Healthy Cities

The growth of health promotion as a topic for discussion and a principle for practice is widespread, and affects all groups of health professionals. The Healthy Cities project, like Health for All, was inaugurated by the World Health Organization and has informed policy throughout the world.

Healthy Cities: Research and Practice examines the application of the project in a number of countries. The contributors explore problems in the relationship between policy-makers, communities and academic researchers, and discuss how the Healthy Cities programme affects housing and health policies, community development, scientific interchange and health education. In addition, the editors, John Davies and Michael Kelly, provide a conceptual framework by tracing the history of the WHO projects and discussing them in the broader context of scientific and philosophical debates about modernism and post-modernism.

The contributors are practitioners and scientists with wide experience in this area from the United Kingdom, Canada, Australia and the United States. *Healthy Cities* will be invaluable to all those working at community level and in government with an interest in health, as well as to students on health promotion courses.

John K. Davies is a former Vice-President of the International Union for Health Education and consultant with the World Health Organization. He is currently Head of Health Promotion with Plymouth Health Authority. **Michael P. Kelly** is Professor of Social Sciences at the University of Greenwich.

Also available from Routledge

Health Promotion: Disciplines and Diversity
Edited by Robin Bunton and Gordon Macdonald

Researching Health Care: Designs, Dilemmas, Disciplines
Edited by Jeanne Daly, Ian McDonald and Evan Willis

Quality and Regulation in Health Care: International Experiences
Edited by Robert Dingwall and Paul Fenn

Healthy Cities

Research and practice

Edited by John K. Davies and Michael P. Kelly

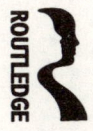

London and New York

First published 1993
by Routledge
11 New Fetter Lane, London EC4P 4EE

Simultaneously published in the USA and Canada
by Routledge
29 West 35th Street, New York, NY 10001

Typeset in Bembo by Michael Mepham, Frome, Somerset
Printed and bound in Great Britain by
Mackays of Chatham PLC, Chatham, Kent

British Library Cataloguing in Publication Data
A catalogue record for this book is available from the British Library.

Library of Congress Cataloging in Publication Data
Healthy cities: research and practice/edited by John K. Davies and
Michael P. Kelly.
   p.cm.
   Includes bibliographical references and index.
   1. World Health Organization. Healthy Cities Project.
   2. Urban health–Research. 3. Urban health–Planning.
   I. Davies, John K. (John Kenneth) II. Kelly, Michael P.
   RA566.7.H434 1993
   362.1'09173'2–dc20 92–45837
                                     CIP

ISBN 0–415–07791–5 (hbk)
      0–415–07792–3 (pbk)

Contents

Illustrations

Contributors

Lee Adams is Director of Health Promotion with Sheffield Health Authority, England.

Frances Baum is Director of the South Australian Community Health Research Unit and Associate Professor in the School of Medicine at Flinders University.

Bruce Charlton is Lecturer in Public Health, University of Newcastle upon Tyne, England.

Lisa Curtice is Research Fellow in the Research Unit in Health and Behavioural Change at the University of Edinburgh, Scotland.

John Davies is Director of Health Promotion, Plymouth Community Services NHS Trust, England, and was formerly Director of Research at the Scottish Health Education Group, Edinburgh, Scotland.

Ron Draper is a freelance consultant for WHO Europe based in Copenhagen, Denmark.

Beverly Flynn is Professor in the Department of Community Health Nursing, Indiana University School of Nursing, and Director of Healthy Cities Indiana, Indianapolis, USA.

Trevor Hancock is a public health consultant in, Kleinberg, Ontario, Canada, and Associate Professor in the Faculty of Environmental Studies at York University, Toronto, Canada.

Sonja Hunt is a freelance health research consultant and board member of the Right to Warmth Campaign, Scotland; she was formerly based with the Research Unit in Health and Behavioural Change at the University of Edinburgh, Scotland.

Michael Kelly is Professor of Social Sciences at the University of Greenwich, London, England, and was formerly Senior Lecturer in Health Promotion in the Department of Public Health at Glasgow University, Scotland.

James McEwen is Professor of Public Health at Glasgow University, Scotland.

Sarah McGhee is Lecturer in Health Services Research in the Department of Public Health at Glasgow University, Scotland.

Michel O'Neill is Professor in Medical Sociology, Community Health and Health Promotion in the School of Nursing at Laval University in Quebec City, Canada.

Jan Smithies is a freelance consultant in health promotion based in London, England.

Agis Tsouros is WHO Healthy Cities Project Officer in Copenhagen, Denmark.

Margaret Whitehead is a freelance health policy analyst based in Shropshire, England.

Foreword

I am very pleased with and encouraged by the growing interest in Healthy Cities research. This is a long-neglected and yet highly needed area of activity. Healthy Cities has become the local level testing ground for what we preach in Health for All, health promotion and the new public health.

Research is needed to assess health needs, to develop practical instruments for public health work and to evaluate the project's multiple macro and issue/activity facets. The strategy, Health for All, was launched nearly a decade ago. Health inequalities, community participation and inter-sectoral work represent key strategic areas that require analytic, qualitative and action-oriented approaches to monitor and evaluate process and outcome. Community and environmental diagnosis methods and tools need to go beyond traditional epidemiology and cover Healthy Cities aspects such as social support, perception of well-being, access to services and special needs of under-privileged groups. Thus it will be possible to create a more credible base for project indicators, city health plans and mechanisms for accountability for health.

The challenge for research institutions and researchers is to mobilize resources, to develop new incentives and, above all, to promote and encourage new approaches for more timely and action-oriented research in project applications.

There is a lot of food for thought and a wide range of good ideas in this publication. I wish to congratulate John Davies and Mike Kelly on their timely initiative.

Ilona Kickbusch, Ph.D.
Director, Lifestyles and Health
WHO Regional Office for Europe

Preface

Our book draws together a range of writers from research and practical backgrounds who have been involved with the Healthy Cities movement and the new public health. These authors provide insights into their various experiences, and, in particular, some of the great difficulties involved in doing work which attempts to break down barriers. The Healthy Cities concept is indeed about breaking down barriers or, in the jargon, working intersectorally. It is about breaking down barriers between local and national organisations (health and otherwise) which provide services to communities. It is also about breaking down barriers between providers and users, such that users have a distinctive voice in, and a good deal of control over, the kinds of services that are provided for them. It is also about breaking down barriers between academic researchers with an interest in health, service provision and social problems and the ordinary men and women about whom, and on whom, such research is conventionally done.

Very many people helped to bring this publication to fruition: Stanley Mitchell, then Director of the Scottish Health Education Group; Professor Donald Campbell, then Dean of Medicine of Glasgow University; David Asquith of the Chief Executive's Department of Strathclyde Regional Council and Sir Thomas Thomson of Greater Glasgow Health Board all provided resources. So, on a smaller scale, did the British Sociological Association's Medical Sociology Group. Our appreciation must also be recorded to the unstinting and generous support of The Healthy Cities Office in Glasgow. We would also like to thank Elizabeth Tribe, Andrew Lyon, Fiona Toal, Catherine Smith, Marion Lacey, Helen Brownlee, Dr Boyd Moir, Sally Daghlian, Dr Alan Barr, Pamela Bartlett, Professor George Forwell, Iain Campbell, Dr Phil Hanlon, Professor Jim McEwen, Drs Carol and Andrew Tannahill, David Black, Dr Graham Watt, Aine Kennedy, Dr Erika Wimbush, Mairi McMenamin and Tessa Kelly. Roz

Lipsey typed the manuscript with her usual exemplary speed and good humour, and Norah Adams provided clerical support throughout. For all their support and assistance we are very grateful and we hope their, our authors' and our own efforts have not been in vain as we move towards healthier cities in the new millennium.

John K. Davies and Michael P. Kelly
Edinburgh and Glasgow

Chapter 1

Healthy Cities
Research and practice
John K. Davies and Michael P. Kelly

THE TENSIONS BETWEEN RESEARCH AND PRACTICE

This book is concerned with the way research relates to practice in the movement known as Healthy Cities and will therefore be of direct interest to those concerned with health policy, health promotion, community development and the reorientation of services towards the community. The main theme of our book is that there is an inherent tension between research and practice in Healthy Cities.

The ancient Greeks regarded illness as a disturbance of the natural balance between the internal and external environments of the person, while the Romans made a contribution to public health through the provision of good water supplies, roads and housing. It was not, however, until the nineteenth century that the individual's environmental and living conditions became the focus of medical attention in a scientific and modern way. This came about following the rapid urbanization that took place in the nineteenth century in England and elsewhere at the time of the Industrial Revolution. Workers flocked to urban centres which rapidly became insanitary and polluted by human and factory waste. Eventually, with the development of reliable transport systems, better-off people moved to the outskirts of these areas. Reformers like Chadwick sought to improve the human environment through better water supplies, sewage and housing. This is a story that is well known and frequently told (Briggs 1968; Webster 1990). In many ways, these environments with their public health infrastructures, their transport systems, and their system of harnessing energy were quite unlike any form of human social organization that had existed before on the planet. They were also amongst the most unhealthy environments ever devised.

It was also in the nineteenth century that public health began to include consideration of broader social issues (Wohl 1983). Ross regards public health during the nineteenth century mostly as never moving beyond its 'relatively uncontentious interests in sanitary engineering' (Ross 1991: 35). However, a socially critical public health approach had been advocated elsewhere through, for example, the work of Rudolf Virchow who argued memorably in the 1840s that 'Medicine is a social science and politics are nothing else than medicine on a larger scale' (Ackernecht 1981). It was out of this broad approach that the seeds of socio-ecological models of public health and urban planning were developed. These developments have been well documented in relation to the growth of the Healthy Cities movement (Hancock and Duhl 1986; Ashton 1992).

Nevertheless, in spite of the early broad socio-ecological view, many commentators have noted the continuous dominance of the biomedical model within public health. This approach was strengthened during the period from the 1930s to early 1970s in industrial countries by the shift of resources and power to the hospital and acute-sector services. This bio-medical model was also used by urban planners during the same period, when the common practice was to move people from their homes and decant them into tower blocks or housing estates outside the city, de-stroying communities in the process (Gans 1967).

However, the biomedical model has not gone unchallenged. Since the mid-1970s, grave concern has been expressed world-wide at the seemingly endless resources required by the increasingly high-technology modern medical care. Attempts have been made in many countries to curtail, or at least to control, the costs through value-for-money assessments, clinical audits, income generation and financial management techniques and systems.

At the same time as the critical and questioning chorus concerning high-technology medical care arose, key developments occurred in Canada which were to give rise eventually to the Healthy Cities project. There, the Lalonde Report (Lalonde 1974) used the ideas of Thomas McKeown (1971) who had highlighted the fact that major improvements in health in the nineteenth century were not due principally to medical interventions, but to public health provision. Based on McKeown's ideas, the Lalonde Report suggested that future improvements in health would arise from improving the environment and promoting lifestyles conducive to health. As it transpired, the second of these issues was more in tune with the prevailing biomedical model. Consequently, health education involving individual behaviour-modification techniques was advocated in many countries. Ironically at the same time, fewer resources were devoted to the research and practice of health education itself. Health education was effectively taken under the wing of preventive medicine (Mitchell and

Davies 1985) and its scientific basis was derived uncritically from social psychology and epidemiology. Health education was seen as an intervention, as a form of treatment, and was measured on a before and after basis. As this approach did not consider the wider socio-economic and environmental factors affecting health, it has been extensively criticized for its victim-blaming approach. In the early 1980s, however, work by people such as Hancock and Duhl (1986) and Kickbusch (1987) led to a revised consideration of social models of health based more on environment than on lifestyle.

Another major development during the 1970s was sparked off by the WHO Alma-Ata Conference and Declaration on Primary Health Care which acknowledged formally the role of community participation in health (WHO 1978). The prevailing paradigm underpinning all WHO activities had until then been the 'treatment model', whereby medical expertise and knowledge were exported from developed to developing countries. Alma-Ata set in motion the 'Health for All by the Year 2000' strategy. This development, occurring at the time of the appearance of the Lalonde Report, and questions about the effectiveness of the pervading medical paradigm, together with consumers' interest in their own health, acted as fertile ground for the new public health.

In 1984 the European Office of the World Health Organization called together a multidisciplinary group to discuss, and make recommendations on, the concepts and principles of health promotion. A document on the concepts and principles of health promotion came from this meeting and was extensively disseminated and translated as a discussion paper (WHO 1984). It set out for the first time the WHO definition of health promotion, which led, in 1986, to the Ottawa Conference and 'Ottawa Charter for Health Promotion' (WHO 1986). This underlined a move towards participation and more effective community involvement. A conference had also been held in 1984, entitled Beyond Health Care – Toronto 2000, which sought to focus intersectoral attention on the city and the health of its citizens from these early beginnings.

In 1986, the WHO Healthy Cities project was formally launched. It was seen as 'a means of legitimizing, nurturing and supporting the process of community empowerment' (Tsouros 1990a). It has grown rapidly and has not, unusually, been based on an underlying research tradition. Using community participation as a method, it seeks to reduce inequalities, strengthen health gain, and reduce morbidity and mortality. Its aims are conventional enough, but its method and philosophy mark a decisive shift in ways of thinking about health in urban environments.

The research base for the Healthy Cities approach is therefore, not surprisingly, in its infancy. No single existing academic field can provide the breadth of vision or the scientific theory and methods to cope with these complex issues. It has been observed that it is possible to develop concepts of health that are useful in policy terms, but exceedingly difficult to measure (Flynn 1992). Often it is social processes that are of critical importance in determining the health status of individuals and communities. The key seems to be in the ecological idea of how complex natural systems or processes work in practice (Ashton 1992: 10). Healthy Cities grew not as a research project, but as a practitioner-led activity consisting of a series of local community experiments. The promotion of health in this view must include the adaptation and transformation of social structures that create ill health. People themselves must be empowered individually and through their local communities to take control of their health. The distinctive feature of the idea lies with the processes involved.

Conventionally, in order to attempt to analyse and assess social and political processes as they affect health or indeed other matters, two principles have been brought to bear or have been invoked: the administrative or managerial/technical principle and the scientific principle (Lyotard 1984). In the administrative mode, problems are defined and solved by experts, and solutions are enacted through national or local bureaucratic agencies. In the scientific mode, the ability of the scientific method and research to find new answers to problems is taken for granted and then applied in ways that allow academics to practise their arts. In the case of Healthy Cities, however, neither of the above principles seems to work very well, no matter how many and what sort of experts are brought in. Throughout our volume the problems of applying traditional forms of scientific method to the complexities of Healthy Cities are explored. Science on its own, it seems, cannot be used to solve such complex and multidisciplinary problems as found in the health environment of cities. Therefore, there is a need for a health promotion research where new paradigms can be developed (Duhl 1988). Ashton (1992) comments, for example, that although hard data are important, so too are stories, anecdotes, and anthropological and journalistic reports on who is doing what to whom. WHO/Euro attempted in 1984–5 to establish such a health-promotion research framework and culture (WHO 1985) to encapsulate more qualitative, ethnographic and action research approaches; and to encourage academics to move from their traditional realms and methods of inquiry, both biomedical and social scientific.

As well as describing experimental research projects of theoretical and practical relevance to Healthy Cities, the authors of the following chapters attempt to define and describe the tensions and stresses between the sectors involved – the community, researchers, professionals and their agencies – in relation to their own experiences with Healthy Cities research in various parts of the world. In the final chapter, the editors reconsider the intellectual arguments which relate to the tensions and stresses. The contributors to the volume demonstrate, in a range of settings, what these difficulties and tensions are. The explanation for these tensions, which is explored in the concluding chapter, is that scientific research in the conventional sense is a modern phenomenon. It stems, in other words, from the great advances in knowledge and understanding of natural and social phenomena which grew out of the Enlightenment. Urbanization, the development of contemporary cities, was also a modern phenomenon, as were the attempts by nineteenth and early twentieth century reformers to solve the health problems of the city – they, too, were based on scientific and rational principles. Healthy Cities as a movement, as an idea, in contrast is *post-modern*. It is based on an aesthetic and moral view of health, not a biophysical view of illness (Charlton and Kelly 1992a). It is ecological and environmental and takes positive subjective health as its central focus. It is not individual and does not take pathology as its principal preoccupation. In simple terms, the tensions recorded in this book reflect attempts to apply conventional scientific (modern) ideas to problems which are post-modern. This, we suggest, has important policy implications. We use the terms modern and post-modern here (and throughout) in the sociological sense developed by writers like Lyotard (1984) and Bauman (1992).

THE ORIGINS OF THE BOOK

This book originated out of discussions involving community activists, academics, health educators and others (Kelly 1988). Specifically, the book arose out of a conference held in Glasgow in April 1991. Central to the meeting was the recognition that many social scientists and epidemiologists conduct research which is concerned with some of the principles of Health for All: equity (or inequity and inequalities), participation, social change, public policy, healthy environments, the development of personal skills and the problems of health service delivery. However, in spite of a very large amount of research activity into these and other areas, at least two constituencies who might use such information seldom appear to do so. In particular, the communities on whom so much social scientific research is conducted, the poor and disadvantaged, see little of its results and appear to benefit still less, while the policy-makers at national and local level, not infrequently, give the impression of being oblivious to the results of such scientific endeavour (Oliver 1992).

Under the banner of Healthy Cities, the Glasgow meeting was convened to bring forward the practicalities of intersectoral working between these groups. The planning committee for the conference knew what they did not want to happen. They did not want a gathering where 'experts', self-styled or otherwise, jetted in and delivered papers to a receptive, passive and admiring audience. They wanted, instead, a genuinely participative conference in which focused discussion about particular problems could take place. They wanted, therefore, to devise a format in which this might occur. It was decided to commission a series of papers on themes which seemed to deal with the research-community-policy interfaces. The people who were asked to prepare the papers were selected on the grounds that they had experience of working at these interfaces. Within this broad brief the authors invited were then free to develop their particular theme in whatever way they chose.

The papers were prepared in advance of the conference and dispatched to delegates about a week before the meeting was due to be held. The plan was that all attenders would have the opportunity to read the papers in advance and be able to make any contributions they thought appropriate in workshops on the first day of the meeting. At these workshops a discussant (not the author) would lead the proceedings. The plan was that on the second day each group would report back to a plenary session and, led by a senior scientist from central government, an attempt would be made to pull it all together.

It never really worked like that. In different workshops the community representatives seized the initiative and redefined the agenda in various ways. Rather than coming together in a way which would allow communities, researchers and policy-makers to share, much of what went on was in an atmosphere of mutual misunderstanding and recrimination. By the end of the second day people were still talking to each other, but only just (Kelly 1991).

The authors of the prepared papers were subsequently asked to redraft their contributions in the light of the kinds of comments which had been made, and these revised papers are presented in this volume along with some newly commissioned chapters examining similar issues in Canada, the USA and Australia.

HEALTHY CITIES: A NEW APPROACH

Healthy Cities and its accompanying ideas of Health for All, health promotion and the new public health constitute a major shift in the conceptualization of health. In Healthy Cities and the new public health,

health is expanded out of the biophysical realm into the socio-political domain. The Healthy Cities programme is a political programme which is about a change in power relations in respect of health and illness, and a fundamental epistemological shift in the conceptualization of health itself. Or at least it has the potential to be so. We shall argue that Healthy Cities and the new public health are post-modern movements underpinned by a post-modern, aesthetic and moral view of health rather than a biological or physical definition of illness. The problem which is implicit throughout this volume, and which the exchanges at our conference were a manifestation of, is the fact that locally and nationally based policy-makers, academic researchers and community members have mostly failed to grasp the real shifts in emphasis, theory and practice that the Healthy Cities movement implies. Instead, many commentators and practitioners remain wedded to a conventional (and modernist) view that science can both liberate the human condition and provide legitimation for the political processes of so doing.

The Healthy Cities movement is indeed about liberation – in particular from the inequalities in health and the absence of basic prerequisites for health. Equally, the overriding belief which seems to dominate much thinking about Healthy Cities is that if enough scientific expertise can be gathered, a technical solution to any problem may be found. The organizers of the meeting in Glasgow held much the same view. Implicitly the conference was convened around the notion that a rationalist social science was 'sitting out there' waiting to be applied in ways that could and should be beneficial to the communities that most needed it. If only enough experts, including ordinary people themselves, could be brought together, then a 'solution' would be at hand (Daghlian et al, 1992).

That the organizers were not the first to think this in the Healthy Cities context is illustrated in some of the chapters in this book. Here various examples are provided of attempts, sometimes novel, to provide rational scientific or rational administrative solutions to community involvement, Health for All and Healthy Cities. The sheer difficulty, not to say impossibility of applying rational principles only becomes obvious once the attempt is made to put it into practice, hence our interest in research and practice.

Our volume raises the question, as did the Glasgow conference, of why the application of an apparently rational principle should be so difficult. Why is bringing people from diverse backgrounds, but with a shared set of beliefs in intersectoral working, so hard to put into practice? The answer, we believe, lies in the fundamentally distinct concerns, politically and philosophically, of the Healthy Cities movement. Healthy Cities, we suggest, is not simply the extension of well-tried modern methods and principles. It is not just a straightforward development of what has gone before in terms of the organisation and delivery of health services. It is, instead, a new form of praxis. The failure has been not to recognize this fact and, instead, to continue to work within the same old frameworks of applied social and natural science. The contributors to this volume provide the evidence for this proposition, and in the conclusion we draw the argument together.

THE PLAN OF THE BOOK

Following this introductory chapter, Trevor Hancock addresses, in detail, the definition of the Healthy City and how it relates to the principles of health promotion. The positive and political definition of health – as against the biomedical definition of illness – is described. The emphasis upon processes of advocacy, enablement and mediation is highlighted. The political elements of building healthy public policy, creating supportive environments, and strengthening community action are also documented. In terms of the overall argument of the book, this definition is crucial, for it is the point at which a holistic, integrated, non-discipline-bound and post-modern definition of health as process and activity is made plain. The importance of health as an aesthetic value is stressed by Hancock when he argues that, in terms of health, people should trust their own intuitive knowledge and pay less attention to experts schooled in the biomedical and epidemiological traditions. Hancock makes a compelling case for an intellectually and scientifically integrated and interdisciplinary approach to the problem. He, however, remains within a conventional model of research informing action. On the basis of the elements which he identifies as critical in the process of the Healthy Cities project, he lays out a useful research agenda. Having done that, he outlines some of the characteristics of what that research should be like – much of which has a decidedly post-modern flavour.

In Chapter 3, Agis Tsouros and Ron Draper identify a set of research priorities on the basis of the mid-term review of the Healthy Cities project. The vital political processes underlying the project are highlighted. The ways in which it is important to make links, or break down barriers between activities involving innovation, practical politics and research are emphasized. Given the arguments about modernism and post-modernism, the debate about the role of the political process and the scientific establishment, this is an important statement. The key implementation problem highlighted by Tsouros and Draper is that in many cases the length of time between political acceptance of the project idea and the achievement of real changes in policies and programmes has been longer than expected. In other words, the translation of the idea into practice is not necessarily easy. Cultural, organisational and historical factors have an effect on the implementation process, thus emphasizing the significance of an integrated approach going beyond single disciplines. The significance of a research-driven agenda and of using research is then described by the authors. Tsouros and Draper demonstrate, on the basis of the evaluation of the Healthy Cities project, the nature of the tensions of doing something which attempts to break out of the usual constraints of discipline-bound science in the form of the application of the principles of positive health and health promotion.

In Chapter 4, Lisa Curtice considers the functioning of the Healthy Cities project in Europe in relation to research. She highlights an important tension: while the Healthy Cities project provides a considerable opportunity for research about its philosophy and practice, that research has been very slow to develop. Interestingly, Curtice describes some of the features of a Healthy City intervention in the context of evaluation, and in so doing captures some of the post-modern elements (without calling them that). In Healthy Cities, she says, 'the "intervention" is not sharply defined, takes different forms in different contexts ... [it is impossible] to make sharp distinctions between cause and effect ... Healthy Cities must be conceptualized as one variable (itself changing) which is interacting with a changing scene. Healthy Cities can be thought of as an encounter, or as many encounters: between the philosophy of contemporary health promotion and the constraints and opportunities affecting health work in cities, between an international organisation and local government networks ... between people and groups'. The difficulties of attempting to apply traditional scientific paradigms to such an activity are very clear. Curtice goes on to describe the way the strategy of Healthy Cities was developed and implemented, and the variations in the process of implementation. She tackles the description of the problems of evaluation in a novel way, using fictional anecdotes and debate to great effect. These anecdotes are fictional in only one sense, however. The issues and tensions identified by Curtice are precisely those which many people working directly with Healthy Cities would immediately recognize. Furthermore, the very distinct perspectives which the different academic disciplines bring to Healthy Cities is indicative of the need for an integrated and non-discipline-bound approach – a post-modern approach – to this particular issue.

Chapter 5 is written by two health promotion practitioners, Jan Smithies and Lee Adams, who describe the problems of power relationships in respect of research and evaluation associated with the principles of Health for All. They focus on the concept of *participatory* research. Both Health for All and Healthy Cities take *participation* as a cornerstone of their activities. Conventional, modernist, scientific research does not. In conventional science, ordinary people only participate as subjects or objects of scientific study. Health for All makes a radical departure from this and begins from the premise of *involvement*. While the ideas of participation and involvement may resonate with certain aspects of post-modernist art and culture, the application of this principle in the area of health services and health promotion is much less easy to visualize. Smithies and Adams describe their own innovative activities along with the great difficulties they encountered in implementation. It has been argued, in the context of post-modernism, that in the modern world, science and political power went together and that one of the major roles of science was to legitimize the actions and activities of power holders. Science in the post-modern world has tended to lose this function (Lyotard 1984). What is intriguing about Smithies and Adams' account is the description of what happens when innovative (and post-modernist?) methods are applied in areas where they are *not* marginal to the political processes but confront them directly. Smithies and Adams supply a detailed description of the participative process and the concept of empowerment. The truly distinct nature of this approach to health, as against more usual concepts associated with an administratively and bureaucratically organised service delivered by professionals to a receptive and dependent client group, is made explicit. This is the key point to grasp about the nature of the Healthy Cities movement. It is much more than trying to find a better administrative solution to a bureaucratic problem. Its ethos is neither technocratic nor managerialist. Its ethos is one in which the users or consumers of services are transformed from docile recipients into proactive participants. It is thus in part a consumerist type of orientation. However, since the concept of the consumer implies a market, and since consumer power is itself related to purchasing power, Healthy Cities has to be more than just another version of consumerism. Against this background Smithies and Adams describe the processes of evaluation. They describe two case-studies which demonstrate the difficulties involved.

In Chapter 6, Sonja Hunt examines the role and function of research more generally. Drawing upon her work on damp housing, Hunt questions the modernist assumption that there is and that there should be a link between policy and research. She reminds us that long before Healthy Cities came onto the scene, social scientists often found themselves marginalized. In part this is a confirmation of Lyotard's (1984) argument that never before in history (at least in the Western World) have academics and scientists been freer to speak their minds, and yet never before have so many people taken so little notice of what they had to say! Hunt takes issue with the assumption (which Lyotard and others have identified as a modernist assumption) that research can have a liberating potential. For Hunt, research is more to do with political expediency than with the desire for social justice; she takes up this theme with reference to research on health and dampness. In so doing, she describes some of the problems of both community participation in research and dealing with the power brokers of research. She also addresses the issue of publicizing the findings and translating them into a political issue. What is notable about Hunt's studies is their hard-nosed scientific design. These were double-blind studies using statistical inference. They were not 'soft' or qualitative. The nature of their reception could not, therefore, be accounted for in terms of their oddity compared to conventional work.

Margaret Whitehead examines the product of research in Chapter 7. Conventionally, she argues, scientific research serves scientific purposes. Those purposes may be career advancement, departmental performance, fame, the love of knowledge for its own sake or whatever; the fundamental point about the product of research is that in a very important sense it belongs to the people who did it and/or the people who paid for it. That is the usual model. Whitehead considers the imbalance between the various stake-holders in research with particular reference to community health research. She argues that community development research tends to be outside the scope of mainstream government funding. Whitehead is also concerned about dissemination. She argues that, traditionally, academics tend to communicate with other academics in a closed language unavailable to ordinary people.

Frances Baum reviews the experience of a pilot Healthy Cities project in Australia in Chapter 8. She explores the extent to which the concerns of laboratory-based science may be applied in community settings. What is particularly interesting is that Baum has attempted to work within a community-development orientation while using fairly traditional, albeit, in part at least, qualitative methodologies. She has also used unconventional methodologies, including moving, three-dimensional visual arts. She describes political-pressure-group activity where intersectoral action was required. In general, Baum finds the eclecticism of her approach to have been successful and to have made a positive contribution to the Healthy Cities Project in which she was involved.

In the next chapter Beverly Flynn reviews experience from the USA. She pays particular attention to the cultural context of the USA as a background to understanding the way Healthy Cities developed there. She examines the diversity of models of community health promotion present in that society. She then reviews an action-research model as applied in the Indiana Healthy Cities project. She depicts the purpose of action research in Healthy Cities as providing informed action, changing decision making and applying knowledge to solve community health problems. Several areas of input were studied: leadership development for community health, dissemination of developed leadership, development of action programmes for community health, and involvement of policy-makers in public health and policy change. She reviews her results against these criteria in public policy and involvement in policy-making.

Michel O'Neill describes innovative work of a participatory kind in Canada, which sets out explicitly to build bridges, in Chapter 10. The extent to which developments in Canada set that country apart from developments in Europe is described, particularly some of the innovative actions stemming from government there. O'Neill's main concern is to examine a series of workshops about the problem of indicators of Healthy Cities (or Communities as they are called in Canada). The interesting thing about this is the attempt at praxis, the explicit linking of theory with practice. Using a range of sociological and anthropological methods, O'Neill describes the processes as he saw and participated in them. Despite Canada's favourable cultural environment, and in spite of previous practical experience, O'Neill reveals tensions and difficulties in intersectoral action. In the final analysis, O'Neill argues that these processes are not only complicated, they are riven by conflict. This he sees as the consequence of a plurality of perspectives and agendas. He concludes that academics are used to defining and dominating knowledge development. Health promotion, he notes, invites academics to play a different role which he defines with reference to social relevance and usefulness. This is part modern and part post-modern. It is post-modern in so far as it sees a new and different role, modern in so far as the criteria for success are based on social relevance.

In Chapter 11, Sarah McGhee and Jim McEwen examine the evaluation of a pilot Healthy Cities project in Glasgow. In one of the city's peripheral housing schemes, inter-sectoral bureaucratic co-operation has been matched at community level by, amongst other things, the mobilization of community health volunteers, providing health information for local residents, and facilitating self-help. McGhee and McEwen describe the methods used to evaluate these activities. Some of the advantages and opportunities presented in such an evaluation are described. From the overall perspective of our volume, two very interesting ironies stand out in respect of the description. First, McGhee and McEwen describe how the evaluative methods involved basic Health for All principles like community participation. They also describe some of the difficulties resulting from this approach. Second, and paradoxically, they describe how the expectations of the community were raised to such an extent that the community members who had become involved as volunteers, expected almost instant concrete results. They note, 'While [volunteers] could see the worth of process measures which assisted them in improving the day-to-day operation of the project, they also wanted to be able to measure improvements in health outcomes or such variables as the number of people in the community eating healthier diets compared with previously'! A positivistically inclined proponent of the medical model could not have more straightforward aims! This raises the important issue that, while the philosophy of Health for All, Healthy Cities and the new public health sets itself apart from the medical model and espouses a kind of new science which occupies a moral high-ground because of its commitment to the community, perhaps the community are not quite as advanced in their thinking and cling to more conventional models of science.

Chapter 2

The Healthy City from concept to application

Implications for research

Trevor Hancock

INTRODUCTION: HEALTH PROMOTION AND HEALTHY CITIES

The Healthy Cities concept is both an old and a new one: old in as much as people have been striving to make cities healthier since the dawn of urban civilization, new in its manifestation as a major vehicle for health promotion – the new public health – in the pursuit of achieving Health for All.

This chapter outlines some of the major elements implicit in the Healthy Cities concept and how they have been applied, and their implications for research. The conceptual elements are divided into two broad categories: concepts about health and concepts about strategies for achieving it. The three key elements relating to health are a positive model of health, an ecological model of health and a concern with health inequalities. The major elements concerned with strategies focus on process, public policy and community empowerment.

The Healthy Cities project should be seen and understood within the context of health promotion, which has been defined in the 'Ottawa Charter for Health Promotion' as 'the process of enabling people to increase control over, and to improve, their health' (WHO 1986).

This definition identifies health promotion as a process that is concerned with empowerment. Furthermore, the concept of health that is used is 'a positive concept emphasizing social and personal resources as well as physical capacities'. According to the 'Ottawa Charter', health should be understood as 'a resource for everyday life' which allows an individual or group 'to identify and to realize aspirations, to satisfy needs, and to change or cope with the environment'. The 'Ottawa Charter' placed great emphasis upon the processes of advocacy, enablement and mediation and upon strategies to build healthy public policies, create supportive environments, strengthen community action, develop personal skills and reorient health services. The Healthy Cities project was conceived as a means of taking these broad concepts and strategies and applying them at the local level, following, in essence, the environmental dictum of thinking globally and acting locally. The startling and unanticipated success of the Healthy Cities project (Tsouros 1990b) is an indication of the power of the concept on the one hand and the readiness – indeed the demand – for such a concept on the other.

To some extent, the rapid take-up of this project and its application in cities, towns and even villages throughout the industrialized world has been a problem – a failure of success – because practice has outstripped theory and research. As DeMarco (1990) notes, health promotion grew out of a critique of practice, not a critique of theory. Health promotion practitioners (and they mostly are practitioners) have been primarily concerned with the failure to promote health adequately and the need for changes in policy, programmes and activities so as to more effectively enhance health. The Healthy Cities project has been very much in that tradition, having been taken up mainly by community-level activists, be they politicians, civil servants or community members. Academic thinking and research has not been a central part of health promotion in general, and in particular the Healthy Cities projects. Thus, five years into the project, there is a lack of good research in the area of Healthy Cities. In part this is because people involved in Healthy Cities projects are interested in action rather than research; in part it is because health promotion and the Healthy Cities concept between them provide some fundamental challenges to the dominant research paradigm and establishment, which will be discussed below. First, however, concepts about health and concerns about health promotion strategies and the implications for practice and research will be examined.

CONCEPTS ABOUT HEALTH

There are three aspects of the concept of health that are implicit, and to some extent explicit, in the health promotion and Healthy Cities models. The first is that health is a positive concept, not merely the absence of disease. The second is that the model of health is holistic or ecological, taking into account all the many different factors that determine health. The third is a particular concern with inequalities in health. Each of these will be reviewed in turn.

A positive model of health

The positive model of health is rooted in the WHO definition of health as 'a state of complete physical, mental and social well-being and not merely the absence of disease or infirmity' (WHO 1946). This means that any assessment of health, be it on an individual or collective basis, cannot be premised upon the measurement of mortality and morbidity. This has of course long been recognized by those in public health, but in practice they still rate countries and cities on the basis of such measures as life expectancy and infant mortality. Measures of morbidity are more difficult to come by, and there has been little standard application of such measures as 'health expectancy' (Wilkins and Adams 1983). Of even less relevance is the ratio of physicians or hospital beds to population, statistics still frequently cited in publications of city rankings (see for example, Marlin *et al.* 1983; Bayless 1983).

One of the challenges this seems to pose is the need to educate the public and politicians alike that there is more to health than death and disease – and that doctors and hospitals are not a major determinant of health status! Interestingly though, when people are asked to talk about what being healthy means to them, and what makes for a healthy community, they do not talk about the absence of disease nor about medical services: this suggests that the problem is not so much one of educating the public, but encouraging them to trust their own intuitive knowledge and to pay less attention to expert compilation of data.

The health of a city and its citizens need to be assessed in terms of their physical, mental and social well-being or fitness (Cappon 1990) as much as, if not more than, their mortality and morbidity rates. Unfortunately, there is as yet no widespread agreement on what those measures should be. The data do not for the most part exist (and certainly not at the local level), and simple, cheap and effective methodologies for assessing physical, mental and social well-being and fitness at the local level are not readily available.

Here, then, is one challenge for research, namely to develop and apply positive measures of the physical, mental and social well-being and fitness of individuals and small populations based on their own experience. These measures need to pay at least as much attention to subjective as to objective assessments of well-being.

An ecological model of health

An ecological model of health – or socio-ecological model of health – such as that shown in Figure 2.1 is also fundamental to health promotion and the Healthy Cities concept. It recognizes that the determinants of health are multifactoral, incorporating both physical and social environmental determinants from the individual level to that of our culture and the global ecosystem. Clearly, as such a model indicates, the determinants of health are far more than simply the provision of hospital and medical services. Rather, health is determined by a broad range of public policies (including those aspects of private corporate practices that have public impact), not only at the national, but also at the local level. Indeed, it is this recognition that is central to the notion that local governments can and must play an important role in enhancing health and well-being, as Parfitt notes: 'Many would be surprised to learn that the greatest contribution to the health of the nation over the past 150 years was made, not by doctors or hospitals, but by local government' (1987).

While this is widely understood by public health practitioners, it is not widely understood or appreciated much beyond the public health sector. Thus one of the first obstacles that has to be overcome in developing and implementing a Healthy Cities project is the reaction by many involved in local government that a Healthy Cities project is, or ought to be, about health services. In fact, one reason for being unwilling to participate in a Healthy Cities project is that local politicians may feel it is an attempt by higher levels of government to 'dump' health care responsibilities (and costs!) on them. None the less, cities that do adopt and implement a Healthy Cities project have recognized and accepted a socio-ecological model of health and have begun to develop and implement a wide range of policy and community activities based on such a model, which will be discussed below.

The implications of a socio-ecological model of health for the research community include the development of a salutogenic epidemiology, that is to say an epidemiology of the causation of good health that can also assess the relative power of different determinants of health and the projected or actual impacts upon health of salutogenic interventions. The term 'salutogenesis' is taken from Antonovsky (1984), who was searching for an understanding of why it was that some individuals survive or remain relatively well in situations where others do not. He thus became interested in what he called salutogenesis as the opposite of pathogenesis. Clearly, there are many salutogens, but equally clearly some are likely to be more powerful than others. The most fundamental salutogens are of course such basic human needs as food, shelter, clean water, a safe environment and peace, a set of factors that are met almost entirely for the citizens of the Western industrialized cities, but are still lacking for many who live in the

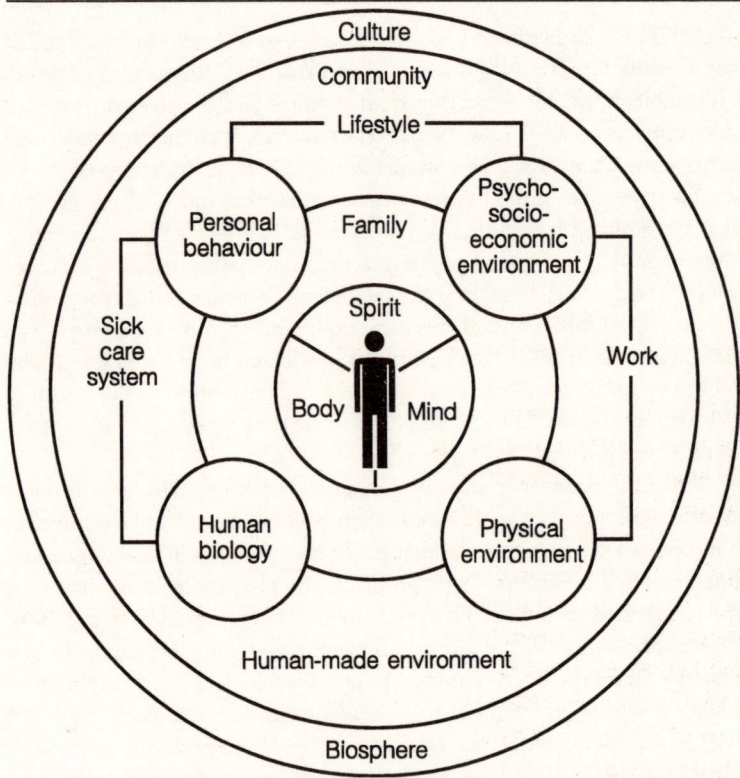

Figure 2.1 The mandala of health: a model of the human ecosystem
Source: Hancock 1985

cities of the less developed nations. But beyond these basic human needs, what are the other significant salutogenic factors? How important are social networks, a sense of self-esteem, power and control over the events and conditions of one's life, income, a sustainable ecosystem and so on? These questions are of great importance, because answering them enables us to decide on appropriate public policy responses. For example, if early childhood development programmes enhance children's self-esteem, producing higher literacy levels and better job prospects resulting in an improved work record, less work strain and less heart disease, then clearly early childhood development could be viewed as (and perhaps funded as) a heart-disease-prevention programme. At present, we are not really in a position to answer those types of questions.

Another implication for research is that if an ecological model of health is used, research needs to be of an interdisciplinary nature; clearly, health researchers acting alone do not have the necessary knowledge base or research skills to address the broad range of determinants of health that the socio-ecological model implies.

Inequalities in health

As a strategy for achieving Health for All, health promotion is vitally concerned with inequalities in health and with means of improving the health of the least healthy in our society. Because inequalities in health are rooted in inequities in access to basic prerequisites for health, health promotion is concerned with social inequity – it is thus not value-free, but on the contrary it is value-laden, socially and politically aware. These characteristics are equally true of the Healthy Cities project. Inequity was the theme of the annual Healthy Cities Symposium in Zagreb in 1988 (Health Promotion 1989) and the theme of inequalities in health and inequities in access to the basic determinants of health has been an important one for project cities. Some of their experience is summarized in the mid-term review of the WHO project (Tsouros 1990b).

Dealing with inequalities in health presents a number of problems for cities. The first is simply whether adequate data exist at the city level to document inequalities in health within the city. The second, and more important, is whether the city has the power and jurisdiction to implement measures that address inequity in access to basic determinants of health. Cities often have powers to confront some of the symptoms of those inequities, but they frequently lack the power to deal with the fundamental economic and social determinants underlying such problems as unemployment, the helplessness and dependency of welfare or the malnutrition and inferior education associated with poverty. The larger determinants of inequity usually lie at the national or international level, and here cities have little or no involvement. However, in those areas where they lack power, cities can and must advocate to national governments (preferably in conjunction with other cities) policy changes that will address the basic determinants of health, reduce health inequalities and improve the health and well-being of their citizens.

There are several implications for research. One, already considered, is the need to tease out the most important determinants of health, and to demonstrate how inequity is related to health inequalities. A second is the need for reliable, cheap and easy-to-apply methods of assessing health status and health determinants at the small-area level. This is so that inequalities in health and inequities in access to health can be documented and monitored at the local level and comparisons made between different neighbourhoods in the city. A third need is for interpretive-qualitative, ethnographic and case-study research on how people experience inequalities in health and inequities in their ability to obtain the basic determinants of health (Kelly 1992). Such research, because it personalizes the experience of our neighbours, often has a more powerful impact than reams of statistics. As McKnight (1985) has remarked, while institutions learn from studies, communities learn from stories. Finally, research is needed on the impact of measures taken to correct inequity in access to basic determinants of health; the results in terms of both subjective and objective physical, mental and social well-being need to be documented, preferably over the short, rather than the long term, since politicians and other funders want to see results from their policies within a short-term (2–3 years) timeframe.

THE PROCESS

Reflecting the emphasis within health promotion upon process, a healthy city has been defined as, 'one that is continually creating and improving those physical and social environments and expanding those community resources that enable people to mutually support each other in performing all the functions of life and in developing to their maximum potential.' (Hancock and Duhl 1986). Thus, it has been clear right from the start that a healthy city is not simply one that has the highest health status but one that is engaged in an ongoing process at multiple levels, from the policy and environmental level down to the individual level, with endeavours at all levels intended to improve health and well-being.

Three particular areas of concern and interest, from an action and research point of view, are those related to the recognition of the project as a process and the public policy and community participation aspects of that process. Each of these three will be considered in turn.

The project as a process

The centrality of process in health promotion and the focus on the Healthy Cities project as a process is axiomatic. Process has been a major emphasis of the evaluation to date; a central component of the mid-term review of the project focuses on what makes for a successful Healthy Cities project (Tsouros 1990b). The emphasis is almost entirely upon process and on structures that support process (Table 2.1). However, this emphasis on process is a problem: since people are accustomed to seeing concrete outcomes, they want status information and they want short-term results.

Table 2.1   Characteristics of a successful Healthy Cities project

Strong political support
Effective leadership
Broad community ownership
High visibility
Strategic orientation
Adequate and appropriate resources
Sound project administration
Effective committees
Strong community participation
Intersectoral collaboration
Political and managerial accountability

Source: Tsouros 1990b

But the process of making a city healthier does not produce quick and easily measurable results, which may make the project difficult to defend.

The implications for research are obvious: research needs to focus on the process of creating a healthy city, so as to inform us about what works and what does not. Some of that research should provide us with answers about short-term changes, since we need to meet demand for short-term measures of impact; but in addition, the research must focus on the long-term development and implementation of processes for health promotion in the cities.

Another implication for research, implicit in what has been said, is that the process of research itself should be examined. Questions need to be raised about the method employed in research, the people who are carrying it out, who is defining the problem and who is receiving and interpreting the results. Healthy Cities research should itself enable citizens to increase control over and improve their health.

Healthy public policy

The strategy of developing healthy public policies is fundamental to health promotion and the Healthy Cities project. A recognition of the important role of local government in establishing the conditions for health has placed a particular emphasis on the need for health-promoting policies in all sectors of local government (Evers, Farrant and Trojan 1990). Thus an important focus for all city projects is the establishment of intersectoral mechanisms and structures that allow different departments within city government (and major sectors beyond city government) to work collaboratively to address the determinants of health in the city.

There are a number of problems with the application of this approach, not the least of which are problems related to vested interests and internal conflicts. However, experience has shown that the concept of health can provide a useful strategic umbrella beneath which a number of different city departments can work collaboratively towards a common goal. However, one of the problems that departments face is in assessing the potential or actual health impacts of various proposed or implemented policies.

In terms of research implications, in addition to the already mentioned need for research on the process, which of course includes the policy-making process, there is a need for models that enable us to assess the possible health impacts of various policy options as well as mechanisms to assess the actual impacts of policies once implemented. These impacts will need to be assessed in terms of health as broadly defined, taking into account physical, mental and social well-being and fitness and both objective and subjective health.

Strengthening community action

In addition to its emphasis on policy, health promotion has a strong emphasis on community action. The definition of health promotion is deliberately vague in talking about 'enabling people' – people here can mean either individuals or groups. As the 'strengthening community action' strategy indicates, we need to enable not only individuals but also communities to become empowered; indeed, it is much more likely that collective action will affect policy than will individual action.

Thus it is not surprising to see a strong emphasis within the Healthy Cities project on community development, community mobilization and community action. The mid-term review of the WHO project suggests varying success in mobilizing community action and enabling the community to become empowered. Given the strong bureaucratic element in every Health Cities project, (resulting from the emphasis on local government) obvious problems arise in getting bureaucracies to accept that communities need to become empowered and that city government must actively enable them to do so. Some communities have been very successful in this regard, with strong and active community participation and leadership in the Healthy Cities project. Other communities, however, have been much less successful in allowing, never mind encouraging, community ownership and community control of the Healthy Cities project. The balance between local government initiative and community initiative is a difficult one to strike.

There are a number of implications for research. The first is the need for good research on the process of community empowerment – what makes for successful community empowerment and what works against it (for that matter, what is community empowerment and how do we measure it?). A second implication is that research should itself be sensitive to the issue of community empowerment: action or participatory research strategies should be utilized so that the community is fully involved in defining the research problem, developing the research model, conducting the research, and analyzing and interpreting it. Another implication for research noted earlier is the need for interpretive or ethnographic studies which allow individuals and communities to tell their own story.

CONCLUSION

Three concluding points need to be made. The first is that we still lack a battery of indicators for the Healthy City. While there has been some agreement that we need a relatively limited number of indicators that are holistic, subjective as well as objective, focus on both process and status, are relatively easy to collect and use at both the city and small-area level, and carry social and political punch, there has been little or no agreement on what those indicators should be. From time to time, lists of indicators have been proposed, but they are always subject to considerable criticism. Indeed, we have been warned about 'the perils of the search and the paucity of the find' (Hayes and Manson-Willms 1990). It may well be that each city will have to develop its own set of indicators to meet its own unique needs, and that we will not be able to develop a set of broadly agreed upon indicators that allow international and intercity comparison; indeed, there is a strong argument that we should not be encouraging between-city comparisons, but rather within-city comparisons. None the less, the indicators issue has not been resolved and will not go away. It will continue to be a matter of much debate not only within the research community but among all who are involved in the Healthy Cities project and would like to be able to assess its relative merit and impact.

The second point is the question that was posed by John DeMarco: 'Knowledge for what?' (and, one might add, for whom?) (DeMarco 1990). Research on and for Healthy Cities, arising as it does out of the value-laden health promotion movement, is not an abstract or pure form of research. It is research with a purpose, it is applied research. It should give us answers that enable us to enhance the health and well-being of people and cities. It should at the same time be an empowering form of research, enabling people to increase control over and improve their health.

Finally, to return to an issue raised at the beginning of the chapter, the implications for research on the application of the Healthy Cities concept include the need for research to be:

- salutogenically oriented
- subjective as well as objective
- concerned with physical, mental and social well-being and and fitness
- holistic
- interdisciplinary
- socially concerned and aware
- concerned with process as much as with outcome
- enabling and empowering
- policy relevant
- interpretive
- action oriented
- community controlled.

Such an approach to research in general runs counter to the dominant research paradigm and the processes of peer review, funding and publication that are controlled by the scientific elite (Lincoln 1990). Health promotion and Healthy Cities researchers will therefore need to address the power structures of the scientific elite if they are to be truly effective. Thus Healthy Cities research is not only about the Healthy City movement, it is fundamentally concerned with the nature and business of health research as we approach the twenty-first century. That is the ultimate implication of health promotion and the Healthy Cities concept for research.

Chapter 3

The Healthy Cities project
New developments and research needs
Agis Tsouros and Ronald A. Draper

INTRODUCTION

In this chapter the findings of the mid-term review of the Healthy Cities project are considered. These findings help to identify a series of research priorities which are subsequently highlighted. The background to the development of the evaluation provides the starting point for the chapter.

THE RESEARCH NEEDS OF THE HEALTHY CITIES PROJECT

By 1988, Healthy Cities looked more promising as a concept than as a practical reality. However, the late 1980s saw the development of the partnerships that have given it more secure foundations. The long-term commitment that has been sustained in a number of cities has paid off in a number of ways, including better methods of municipal government and policies and practices that contribute to the health of city inhabitants.

Perhaps the most important initial gain has been the interest and creativity that has been generated among political leadership in many European cities and indeed in other parts of the world. Health has become much more visible on the political agenda of many cities, regardless of developments at national level in individual countries, and practical understanding of policies that promote health has been broadened. Along with this has come the successful accumulation of practical knowledge about the organizational structures and management strategies that are needed to put Healthy Cities ideas into practice. It is now possible to prepare a composite picture of the arrangements that predict success in taking new approaches to public health at the local level.

The starting point for the Healthy Cities project was the recognition that cities have a significant role to play in promoting health and they are in a unique position to implement public health measures that reflect current thinking about ecology and the environment. The Healthy Cities concept is indeed a recipe for quality living in an urban environment. Cities should, according to the Healthy Cities philosophy, provide a clean and safe physical environment of a high quality based upon sustainable ecosystems. They should offer their inhabitants access to the prerequisites for health (food, income, shelter) – and a wide variety of experiences based upon a diverse, vital and innovative economy. All of this should occur against the background of local historical and cultural factors. Spreading this understanding of Healthy Cities philosophy was one of the fundamental aims of the WHO project.

The WHO project is specifically political and process-oriented in its approach. It pursues its goals by promoting political commitment and advocating fundamental change in local municipal institutions and their relationship with the community and its inhabitants. Cities' policies are examined for their impact on health. The end-point of the project is to be innovative action that promotes equity, sustainable and supportive environments, active community participation in city activities and, ultimately, better health for people who live in cities.

By 1991, WHO was working with a network of thirty project cities located throughout Europe, but mostly in the western part of the region. There were also eighteen national Healthy Cities networks in the region that were linked to the WHO project. Many of the cities in the WHO network have been instrumental in establishing national networks. The activities of the project are based on strategies that have been developed and endorsed by the cities that are in the network. Examples include the planning framework for the 1988–92 period (WHO 1988), the information and exchange strategy used by the project and the Multi-City Action Plan. Perhaps the strongest indication of collective political commitment to the project is the Milan Declaration adopted by mayors and senior politicians from most of the network cities in 1990. Seven strategic priorities for the 1990s are identified. They are:

1 To increase the number of cities in the network from thirty to forty. Most of the new cities will be in Central and Eastern Europe, countries that are under-represented in the project as it now stands.
2 To implement the thirteen Multi-City Action Plans already agreed and to establish processes for their evaluation. The plans are based on arrangements through which cities come together to address common concerns and find practical solutions in areas such as care of the elderly, programmes for youth, mental health, AIDS, and housing.

3 To complete the second round of consultation and evaluation leading to a status report for the first five years of the project running from 1986 to 1991. Such a report was released at the Healthy Cities Symposium held in Copenhagen in June 1992.
4 To decentralize several of the support activities originally performed by the WHO project office, taking advantage of the knowledge and experience that project cities have accumulated. Through this, WHO would build on the strength of cities to expand the capacity of its project office in areas such as consultation, training, technical advice and project evaluation.
5 To support the growth of national networks in Central and East European countries and promote exchange of experience between those new networks and the ones that have existed for some time in the western part of the region.
6 To develop a strategic framework for the next planning period reaching from 1992 to 1995.
7 To support globalization of the Healthy Cities idea by working with the WHO project office being established in Headquarters. The technical discussions at the 1991 World Health Assembly dealt with health and urbanization and were based to a large extent on Healthy Cities experience.

Healthy Cities was from the outset a self-conscious, innovative project that attempted to develop new ideas in public health and the management of municipal enterprises. Because of its innovative nature and the challenges it posed to many assumptions and practices in public health, research was an essential ingredient for the long-term success of the project. It has been agreed that Health for All, health promotion, Healthy Cities and the new public health all require new and creative approaches to research (Kelly 1989). This is expressed as a demand for research projects that are systematic and comprehensive, practical and applied and qualitative. Such projects should focus on policy development, organizational behaviour, information systems, health impact studies and the development of health indicators. Above all, they should be interdisciplinary. The bridge between innovation and practical politics and research has therefore been an important sub-theme in the project.

Unfortunately, little research has been done that focuses directly on the practical issues that cities have encountered in putting the Healthy Cities philosophy into practice. Not enough new knowledge has been developed on the opportunities for Healthy Cities action, the barriers it must overcome and the structures and processes that make it possible to achieve change in the complex urban environments that are prevalent in Europe. From the point of view of WHO, by 1991 it was important to have moved beyond generalizations to initiating action leading to usable research. This should be of the type that will facilitate political and organizational change. A systematic strategy including a plan of action to achieve four results were therefore identified. This had the following elements:

- It would facilitate closer links and *communication* between decision-makers, health activists and the research community. Out of this communication would come the understanding needed to arrive at an agreed set of research priorities.
- The strategy should enable research institutions to be more *actively involved* in local projects, offering mechanisms for better collaboration reaching up to the national and international levels. National Healthy Cities networks as well as WHO have important roles to play in this. The newsletter concerned with Healthy Cities research that was developed was the first step in this direction (De Leeuw 1990).
- The strategy should provide *incentives* for the research community to undertake cross-departmental and interdisciplinary research projects that meet the priorities of individual cities and the project networks. The first-round evaluation of the WHO project has given us a much clearer picture of immediate research needs.
- The strategy should promote wide agreement on a set of practical and immediate research *priorities*. There are many issues to be covered and it is important for them to be tackled co-operatively.

By 1991 the WHO Project Office had completed its first assessment of the experience of network cities in developing project infrastructure and undertaking innovative health action. The results of this assessment were included in the mid-term report (WHO 1990). The assessment was completed in July 1990. It raised many issues that suggested a need for further research. The assessment process itself brought to the fore several problems that will arise in doing applied Healthy Cities research.

WHO needed the assessment for political as well as managerial processes. Politically, the mid-term report has helped to raise the visibility and credibility of the project and managerially it gave a clearer picture of the structures and processes that contribute to project success. The project office undertook the assessment with three purposes in mind. One was *accountability*, that is, to determine generally the degree of progress that had been made towards the stated aims of the project and the constraints that may have prevented more progress. The second was *support*, that is, to help cities in the WHO network by providing specific policy and managerial advice to each of them, based upon a comparison of their experiences. The third was *knowledge development*, that is, to prepare a systematic picture of the processes being used in local projects, their influence on the city institutions and their contribution to the development of a new public health. This knowledge provides a preliminary basis for resource materials and training.

The WHO analysis covered roughly the first half of the first five-year phase of the project extending from 1986 to 1991. It addressed both process and outcome. It was concerned with process because it examined how political commitment was gained and what kind of organizational structures and managerial processes were adopted to do project work. It was concerned with outcome in the sense that it took up examples of progress made in promoting equity and in dealing with particular lifestyle, environmental and health service problems. In general, cities have made more progress in developing structures and processes than in introducing innovative policies and programmes. In many cities, the length of time between political acceptance of the project idea and the achievement of the real changes in policies and programmes has been longer than expected by both WHO and local practitioners.

The analysis is based on information obtained in questionnaires completed by each of the twenty-five cities in the network at the time the analysis was done and from interviews held with representatives of projects in each city. It is important in examining the results of the analysis and planning research of a similar kind to recognize that the assessment process was developed and refined continuously over the eighteen-month period during which it took place. Towards the end of the project, for example, it became clear that it was essential to visit local people for interviews to gain a clear understanding of how projects worked. At that point interview coverage was extended beyond project staff to include politicians, administrators from municipal departments and, of course, community representatives. This kind of flexibility is essential in exploring the dynamics of innovative initiatives such as this, which, by definition, are going through a process of constant change.

Two products came out of the analysis. One was a consultation report for each of the twenty-five cities that were covered, offering them advice on policy planning and management practices. The other was the mid-term review. Experience gained in the analysis was used to prepare a questionnaire for a second round of interviews. The main conclusions of the initial analysis were:

– Several characteristics of cities have a profound effect on the degree of success that projects achieve and the ways in which they develop. Most significant is the size of the city, the strength and nature of its economy, political preferences and traditions, the way in which municipal administration is organized and the assumptions about community participation in the life of the city and its administration. Cross-national comparisons made these distinctions very obvious.

- Political commitment is essential for project success. Such commitment from mayors and city councillors is needed to raise visibility, public awareness and interest in various sectors, act as an advocate around controversial issues and provide leadership in broadening the understanding of how city policies and practices contribute to health.

- About half of the project cities had developed new organizational strategies for addressing health. These rest upon intersectoral action generated by politicians and senior administrators, local action based in the community and open proactive support coming from well-organized project offices that are able to think strategically. A trend towards decentralization of decision-making was apparent in a number of cities.

- Multisectoral committees that provide political direction for projects, oversee their planning and promote communications amongst organizations that become project partners are essential ingredients in project success. There is now a large body of practical knowledge on finding leadership for intersectoral communities, setting their terms of reference, choosing their membership, planning their agendas and providing the support they need to work effectively. By the same token, it is possible to gain an understanding of the most important constraints on their development in cities with a long tradition of separation and conflict between departments and sectors.

- Project offices function in a variety of ways depending upon the context in which they work. In most cases, they are an important medium for communication and information exchange, a support system for intersectoral committees, a source of new ideas and the mechanism through which community groups gain recognition and support. One of their important roles has been to increase the legitimacy and acceptability of ideas that were previously viewed as somewhat marginal.

- About half a dozen ways in which Healthy Cities projects offered support to community groups were identified. These include provision of technical advice and information, establishing communication networks, helping in the search for financial aid and, in some cases, undertaking straightforward community development. In general, however, there was a lack of long-term strategy for strengthening

community participation. Indeed, absence of strategic thinking was a characteristic of many projects.
– Political and managerial accountability were noted to be weak spots in most projects.

When the analysis was completed, a fairly clear picture of qualities or characteristics that are needed for projects to perform well could be discerned. These qualities are the preconditions for success. They are present to varying degrees in those projects that have achieved significant progress so far. If projects are not working well, a good way to offer help is to determine which of these qualities are missing, why they are absent and what can be done to work towards their achievement. The important qualities are strong political support, effective leadership, broad community control and high visibility. Projects also need to have a strategic orientation supported by adequate resources and sound administration. Co-operation between sectors is essential and a strong accountability maintains long-term links with the political system and the community.

One of the original aims was to document the rich experience of the project so that it could be used to develop tools that could be adopted and adapted by other city administrations. The changes that have taken place in Central and Eastern Europe during the first years of the operation of the project, have created an additional demand for such material and opportunities to use it in the widespread renewal that is taking place. Examples would be urban health profiles, city health plans, and handbooks on health management in the local context, as well as training materials.

An agreed set of research priorities is one of the four elements of an effective Healthy Cities research strategy. The WHO analysis points towards six areas where research is obviously needed. In some cases, research will have to be repeated in a number of cities to provide evidence that will convince politicians and decision-makers in the municipal government and business. In all cases, sharing of results will contribute to the general pool of knowledge about theory and practice that is needed to undertake innovative institutional and policy change.

1 *Equity:* Reducing inequalities in health is a universal Healthy Cities priority. Much more about the health status of the economically and socially disadvantaged and its influence on the quality of their lives needs to be known. What are the consequences of the disadvantages they suffer in terms of access to housing, transport, cleaner environments, education, work and social contacts? What are the attitudes in different cultures to affirmative action on their behalf and how well do affirmative action measures work? Do they have effects that are not anticipated?

2 *Prerequisites for health:* A good deal is already known about the consequences for health that come from poor housing, inadequate food, limited education, prolonged unemployment, poor access to primary care and few opportunities for leisure and recreation. It was surprising to find in the analysis, however, that generalized and scientifically convincing results were not always sufficient to generate political support and action, especially where new costs were involved. It seems to be essential to document the health impact of these disadvantages down to the city, and even the neighbourhood, level. Well-documented research in these areas will be an important precondition for political advocacy and action.

3 *Policy and programme impact:* Because of its commitment to intersectoral action, Healthy Cities is an important leader in the movement towards a new public health. However, not all politicians nor business leaders appear to be convinced about the impact of urban planning and housing policy, traffic and pollution control, development of recreational facilities and improvement of public transport on health. To meet this problem, more investigation of the impact of urban policy on health will be essential. Indeed in many cases, this will have to begin with the development of new concepts and methodology for doing such impact studies.

4 *Intersectoral action:* Intersectoral action challenges traditional patterns of organizations and management in the public sector. Municipal departments are usually organized around specialized sectors of activity with vertical lines of responsibility, running from city council through senior managers to the operational level. Efforts to work across departmental lines frequently encounter political, managerial and professional resistance unless each of these groups can see it as being to their advantage. More research is needed to develop organizational theory and practice to overcome the constraints that these traditions place upon co-operative action between sectors in the interest of health. More information about organizational structures, planning mechanisms, decision-making tools and evaluation methods will foster co-operative action and the sharing of responsibility.

5 *Community participation:* The WHO analysis similarly identifies a number of barriers to community participation in problem definition, planning, decision-making and action in so far as they affected Healthy Cities initiatives. These include differing political cultures, bureaucratic resistance, professionalization of knowledge, and reluctance on the part of individual citizens to become involved. The project will benefit from international comparisons of these various kinds of resistance and the

benefits of new structures and processes that are created to overcome them.

6 *Strategic planning:* Healthy Cities is committed to the development of urban environments that are supportable and sustainable. Health is linked with well-being and to social and cultural development. The concept is ecological, viewing the city as a system and emphasizing the interaction between its various networks. Effective action in this kind of context requires a strategic perspective that is long term and comprehensive, combining a clear sense of direction with the ability to adapt flexibly to changing circumstances. This kind of strategic thinking is relatively new in the field of health and social policy and will demand new planning, theory and methodology. To make Healthy Cities faithful to its promise, it is critical for researchers to make creative contributions in this area.

From WHO's point of view, the Healthy Cities project has laid the basis for a new European public health movement and has brought us directly in contact with local governments, making us more visible and relevant to their concerns. There are few examples in the history of public health, where a relatively small investment has paid off so well. The concepts and principles of Healthy Cities are widely accepted with more than 300 cities in the region identifying themselves with national networks in one way or another. The challenge now is to move from concept to practice. Interdisciplinary research that combines traditional public health with other analytical perspectives and disciplines must be able to contribute to this transition.

Chapter 4

Strategies and values

Research and the WHO Healthy Cities project in Europe

Lisa Curtice

INTRODUCTION

This chapter is based on work which was carried out in co-operation with the Healthy Cities Project Office in Europe to monitor the progress of cities in the early years of the project and which has been reported by Curtice and McQueen (1990) and by Tsouros (1990b). Thirty cities were included in the European project at that time. The formal monitoring of project cities conducted by WHO for the years 1988–9 comprised written annual progress reports and semi-structured interviews. The progress reports were completed in English by workers in project cities and signed by the leading political representative; these produced mainly quantitative information about the state of project development in the participant cities. The interviews were conducted with city project teams, sometimes in the city, but more usually at one of the annual conferences, and were noted, but not recorded verbatim. The four UK project cities (Belfast, Blooms-bury/Camden, Glasgow and Liverpool) were the subject of visits lasting two to three days in 1990 where consultations with a broader range of groups and tours of the city took place. In addition, the Healthy Cities Project Office at WHO/Euro has access to a large amount of informal material, including background information on the cities, local Healthy Cities publicity material, reports and strategy documents and case-studies prepared for presentation at the annual symposia. The Research Unit in Health and Behavioural Change of the University of Edinburgh was invited, as a WHO Collaborating Centre for Health Promotion Research, through the Health Education Board for Scotland (then the Scottish Health Education Group) to assist with the analysis of the two rounds of progress reports and interviews and to take part in some of the 1989 interviews and in all of the UK consultation visits.

It is not suggested that the exercise just described, which was part of the project's mid-term review, represents all the research that has been conducted on Healthy Cities in Europe. WHO/Euro is drawing together all the materials which it has available on cities in the European project to produce a five-year review of progress. Project cities have routine data available to them; in 1989 three-quarters of the project offices reported that they had access to basic data relevant to their project (Curtice and McQueen 1990). There are examples of research commissioned by individual project cities and many examples of research carried out as an integral part of Healthy Cities activities, such as the participatory community health profile in the Blackstaff area of Belfast (Tsouros 1990b). Work continues within the project on the development and implementation of appropriate indicators (WHO Healthy Cities Project 1988a). Research networks and strategies are being developed in the national networks of Healthy Cities, which include cities not in the WHO project (Thunhurst 1989), and there are attempts to create international clearing houses for Healthy Cities research (De Leeuw 1991a). Arguably, however, the mechanisms have not yet been developed for overall evaluation of the project in Europe.

The demands of evaluation must figure in any Healthy Cities research

First Round (1987)	Second Round (1988)	Third Round (1989)
Barcelona, Spain	Belfast, United Kingdom	Dublin, Republic of Ireland
Bloomsbury/Camden, United Kingdom	Copenhagen, Denmark	Kaunas, Lithuania
Bremen, Germany	Eindhoven, Netherlands	Nancy, France
Dusseldorf, Germany	Glasgow, United Kingdom	Seville, Spain
Horsens, Denmark	Gothenburg, Sweden	Frankfurt, Germany
Liverpool, United Kingdom	Jerusalem, Israel	
Pecs, Hungary	Liege, Belgium	
Rennes, France	Milan, Italy	
Sofia, Bulgaria	Montpellier, France	
Stockholm, Sweden	Munich, Germany	
Turku, Finland	Padua, Italy	
	Patras, Greece	
	Vienna, Austria	
	Zagreb, Croatia (then Yugoslavia)	

Figure 4.1 European cities included in the first three years of the WHO Healthy Cities project
Source: Curtis and McQueen (1990)

agenda, yet there is no consensus as to the appropriate methodologies for such a task. The Healthy Cities project in Europe is not a planned intervention which is seeking to demonstrate the efficacy of certain pre-defined approaches to the promotion of health, but rather a relatively high-risk and pluralist enterprise. Cities admitted to the European project have encompassed a wide variation in size, political responsibility and economic status, ranging from metropolitan conurbations such as Barcelona to relatively small towns such as Horsens in Denmark (Figure 4.1). Simple comparisons of activities in such widely differing contexts are unlikely to reveal which approaches have been most successful. There are, however, questions of immediate interest which might be answered at this stage. For example, why, in a variety of demographic, institutional, political and cultural contexts, have health promoters, politicians, technocrats and community groups embarked on a range of health promotion activities under the label of Healthy Cities? What does Healthy Cities health promotion look like in practice? Is it new and, if so, in what way? Why has the idea of Healthy Cities exerted such widespread appeal? It may be wrong to conceptualize Healthy Cities activities as unique or discrete entities. Within project cities it may be inappropriate, therefore, to try to distinguish the contribution of local Healthy Cities projects from other developments, because the projects do not always see themselves as independent actors, but rather, as facilitators. This view was strongly expressed on several of the 1989 progress reports, for example:

> The project is a process in a city with 70,000 employees and 430,000 inhabitants. As the project is integrated into different committees and departments it is not meaningful for us to try and describe the content in the way requested. A lot of activities of the kind that are asked about have been done this year. But they have been done by different committees and departments, and it would not be true to their ambition to make this city a Healthy City, to say that all these activities are the result of the Healthy Cities Project 'Frisha Goteborg'.
>
> (1989 progress report from Gothenburg, Sweden, cited in Curtice and McQueen 1990)

> Everybody who is supporting our project is doing this under the label of the aim of the project. Together we try to reach this aim. Projects are autonomous. They are not established under the umbrella of the Healthy Cities Project ... networking is always on mutual terms.
>
> (1989 progress report Eindhoven, Netherlands, cited in Curtice and McQueen 1990)

Evaluation in the context we have described cannot follow a classical model (WHO Healthy Cities Project 1988c). The intervention is not sharply defined, takes different forms in different contexts and cannot be reduced to discrete components. It may not always be possible or relevant to make sharp distinctions between cause and effect. The important questions are rather, what sorts of action, in what sorts of circumstances are effective. Healthy Cities must be conceptualized as one variable (itself changing) which is interacting with a changing scene. Healthy Cities can be thought of as an encounter, or many encounters: between the philosophy of contemporary health promotion and the constraints and opportunities affecting health work in cities; between an international organization and local government networks; between strategic approaches to improving health in cities and local political needs; between people and groups who had long been working on local health issues or seeing health in a holistic way and new partners; between the time-scale of health promotion strategies and the timing of historical events. The second part of this chapter will be concerned especially with the conditions for one particular encounter: that between research and the developing project. The researcher's is only one of several existing and possible accounts of the project. Three perspectives will therefore be considered here: the official or public account of the project, the perspectives of local city projects and a research perspective drawing on the social sciences.

A EUROPEAN MODEL?

Before discussing a city perspective and one research perspective on the early development of the Healthy Cities project, it is worth while describing the official aims of that project. Evaluation must come to terms with participants' own rationales of their actions, and in this section a summary is presented of the basic premisses of the project, based closely on the statements of key protagonists. This short overview of the terms in which the Healthy Cities strategy has been presented is also important for interpreting the kinds of responses received from researchers, including the response of ignoring the project.

The Healthy Cities project in Europe was established by WHO in 1986 as a demonstration project (WHO 1986b). The operational strategy was for a handful of European cities to transfer the lessons of public health work at city level to other cities, through national and international networks (Dr John Ashton, personal interview, February 1990). There would thus be a ripple effect, with cities acting as agents or message-bearers of a more participative and politically aware public health practice which would put content and detail into the relatively empty boxes of sustainable health policies.

The wider strategy, to which this process of diffusion was intended to contribute, was to make health a major public policy issue throughout Europe. A critical mass of cities, in which health issues were prioritized, was seen as the basis of a powerful and effective new public health lobby. City governments were identified as agents of the new public health movement because, by adopting city health plans, they could demonstrate the value of making health a reference point for public decision-making. They were also perceived by WHO as the level of government best placed to be a focal point for public participation in health (Kickbusch 1989). The political process which Healthy Cities projects were to engage in was coalition-building; consensus, presumably as to the importance of health issues to all groups in the city, was to be the means to keep health on the political agenda.

The Healthy Cities project has developed a vision of what a healthy city could be like. The definition of health underlying the Healthy Cities project in Europe is social and ecological (Tsouros 1990b: 20). The vision of what a truly healthy city would be like includes good health for everyone who lives there and universal access to high quality health services, both public health services and services for those who are ill. These qualities alone, however, do not define a healthy city. People in a healthy city would be living in an unpolluted, safe environment; the built environment, particularly housing, would be of high quality. The city would be supported by, and contribute to, the development of a stable and sustainable ecosystem. Social life would be rich and political participation highly developed. Thus, if you lived in a healthy city you would feel that you were supported by a community in which there was mutuality in human relations and the absence of exploitation. Decisions which directly affected the well-being of individuals would not be taken only by some remote bureaucrat or planner, but would be reached after widespread public debate; decentralization of decision-making would devolve power and give people greater control over the decisions which affected them.

The healthy city would have a diverse and vital economic base. In a healthy city no group would be deprived of the basic resources for life – food, shelter, income, safety, work – and there would be equal opportunities of access to a wide range of cultural and social experiences. Communication between different groups in the city would be encouraged by the political, social and physical form of the city and people in the city would have a strong, but not exclusive, sense of their cultural identities, reinforced by historical awareness of the many components of the city's past (WHO Healthy Cities Project 1988a). Recent developments in Europe have suggested that peace must also be considered a prerequisite for the development of health in urban communities.

To start up a Healthy Cities project involves encouraging the development of processes in the city which will lead to people having healthier lives. There is no set way to go about this. The overall planning framework for the first five years of the European project sets out the main action areas for the project, derived from the 'Ottawa Charter for Health Promotion': pursuing equity, developing community action and individual skills, creating supportive environments, reorienting health services and developing healthy public policies (WHO Healthy Cities Project 1988b). These phrases are shorthand for a number of concepts, some more well developed than others, which form the broad basis for agreement among some health promoters as to the way to improve public health. Projects by themselves will not achieve long-term shifts in the orientation of public policies. Public policy-making agencies must be made to account for the health impact of their policies, and organizational mechanisms of collaboration are needed to ensure that health concerns are taken on board at all stages of policy development and implementation (Milio 1986).

Project cities would have a four-pronged strategy. First, to be selected for the project, the sponsors in the city would have to demonstrate that there was political will to develop a city health plan and to devote resources to the project; in other words, political commitment to the goals of Healthy Cities was a quality essential in project cities. This would also be demonstrated by participation in the European network and taking responsibility for setting up a national network of Healthy Cities (WHO Healthy Cities Project 1988c, Appendix 2: 38). The second element of the strategy was visibility. Third, projects were expected to work on changing the organizational culture of city governments because cross-sectoral health policies are almost impossible to implement effectively within a fragmented bureaucratic structure where there is no established means to enforce public accountability (Tsouros 1990b). Finally, city projects would have to be able to show some short-term gains. They needed to set up or work with a small number of well-defined programmes or projects which were clearly innovative and would demonstrate the value of new approaches to developing health in cities. Short case-studies of specific actions have been presented by city teams at the annual symposia of the European project.

The formal Healthy Cities strategy retained its basic shape as the project moved from a developmental to an implementation phase, although more cities were selected to join the project in response to the very great popularity of the Healthy Cities idea (see Figure 4.1). While an overview of the strategy emphasized the coherence of the project's core values, a mid-term view from the cities presented a picture of considerable variation in the context, status and development of projects. This latter view was the picture presented by the data available at the beginning of the analysis of the project in 1989. The position illustrates the problems in drawing conclusions of evaluative significance without detailed awareness of the history and context of the development of projects in particular cities.

A VIEW FROM THE CITIES

Analysis of the 1989 progress reports showed great variation in the state of development of city projects. Thus the monetary resources devoted to projects, as measured in the annual budget for administering the project office, varied from nothing in a quarter of project cities to $700,000 in others. Measurement of project resources in terms of money budgeted, however, may not have reflected the value of project offices, since not all had separate project budgets. Staffing levels of projects, however, measured in full-time equivalents, suggested that the resources available to projects were relatively modest in 1989. Total staff time ranged up to 4.5 full-time equivalent staff (FTE), but the modal staff for city projects was 1.5 FTE and a third of the cities had less than a half-time co-ordinator. The amount of staff time available to projects was not apparently related to the length of time the city had been in the project, nor to the size of the city in which it was based (Curtice and McQueen 1990).

The semi-structured interviews which had been conducted with project teams, and the comments provided on the open questions in the annual progress reports provided some insights into the variation reported by project cities. Cities entered the Healthy Cities project with very different baselines of political preparation and institutional development. The project in Gothenburg, for example, was located within the Public Health Council (*Halsarat*) which had been established in 1981, following the recommendations of a health promotion committee which had existed since 1975. In some other cities, the orientation to health promotion was much more recent and lacked a developed institutional base. Projects differed in the extent to which they were in fact city-based or were organized, or had key partners at regional or provincial level. Projects could be observed to be developing different emphases, for example in the extent to which they worked openly with the public or adopted a rational or responsive planning strategy (Curtice and McQueen 1990, Section 4; Tsouros 1990b: 63), although these emphases were not determined by the institutional setting. Writing about the uneven progress towards the adoption of Health for All policies by health authorities in the UK, Rathwell (1991) has also pointed to differences in the context of awareness, commitment and organization at local and national level in accounting for the adoption of HFA policies.

A co-ordinated but decentralized evaluation strategy in which information was collected locally would make it possible to provide truly city-centred accounts of the development of the project in Europe. As it is, detailed information about the dynamics of projects within cities is not uniformly available. Visits to the four UK cities in 1990, however, provided a window on the perceptions of those involved in Healthy Cities projects and the difficulties and rewards they faced in their work.

There follows a fictional account from a project co-ordinator, which is illustrative of the shift in the research agenda which would occur if research were to be driven by the developmental needs of the project; an emphasis on process, on organizational developments and on strategic options comes to the fore. Moreover, the account suggests that judgements as to the success of the project at any one time may be as difficult for the practitioner, working on the inside, to make in isolation, as for the researcher or evaluator, on the outside.

The project co-ordinator's mid-term report:

We have spent a lot of energy in the two years establishing the intersectoral group. It has been hard work trying to establish some common ground between the politicians, departmental officials and community representatives, and at times you wonder if it is ever going to get beyond a talking shop. But when we got involved in the pilot project to reduce accidents on a local estate we began to feel that we really had established the personal and organizational links which might make a difference to the outcome of the project. It's hard to explain, but you can see shifts in people's perceptions and you know that there are contacts now between members of groups which never used to talk to each other, and then people start to co-operate in projects and you think: this *is* a process of social change. At other times the project structures seem far more fragile. City politics are dominated by the issue of financial cutbacks and the project seems to be marginalized. A few key individuals switch their attention elsewhere and some of the links between different groups break down. Above all, the gap between the magnitude of the tasks and the resources available can be crushing. It is hard to keep action going on all fronts, to keep media interest alive, to prioritize the issues identified by the steering group and to pursue a long-term strategy of consultation and public involvement.

None the less, some activities are flourishing. When we started, there were a number of groups around who were already working on health issues and who shared quite a lot of our basic concerns, so we got involved with them and now we have a couple of local pilot projects which are really showing the advantages of involving people directly in identifying local health issues. Work on the city health plan is proceeding piecemeal and taking longer than expected, but some good things have emerged. We have representatives from each of the local areas we are involved in on our working groups and one of them has been helping to draft a safety policy. We have drawn up a strategy for community development in health which is going to the health authority, and the elements of a comprehensive health policy for the elderly have emerged from the elderly forum set up by the project which has a membership drawn from health care and social work agencies and carers' groups.

No single perspective will accurately embody the nature of the Healthy Cities project. Evaluation issues are complicated by the variation inherent in the project, by the unevenness of available information and by different levels of research needs. A research perspective is presented below which was developed out of the awareness of these limitations.

A RESEARCH PERSPECTIVE

The perceived significance of the Healthy Cities project as a learning and demonstration project has been affirmed by the decision of the World Health Organisation to extend the funding of the project from five to ten years. This raises the question of the nature and impact of the Healthy Cities phenomenon. The success of Healthy Cities is evidence of the continuing influence of the WHO European Office in setting strategic directions for European health promotion. Preliminary analysis of the early development of the project suggests that the value of an international strategy is to provide a framework within which a range of approaches can be developed and legitimized. Entry-points, structures and issues may have to be locally determined. The experience of the early development of Healthy Cities in Europe also points to the fact that comprehensive strategies may be unevenly implemented. This poses problems for evaluation: it may be misleading to judge the significance of developments in particular contexts against the overall strategy.

It would be justifiable to look to health promotion theory for an explanation of the extremely rapid spread of the Healthy Cities idea in Europe and beyond, but any such attempt would strain the application of diffusion of innovations theory which has such wide currency in health promotion. It may not be entirely helpful to compare Healthy Cities to an innovation, as if it held within it a new technology which could be applied to solve the health problems in European cities. There may be much more analytic value in seeing the healthy city as an important symbol which communicates the message that healthy environments are accessible and politically desirable.

If the Healthy Cities project is conceived as an enterprise to change the way health is perceived, valued and acted upon, a suitable starting point for future evaluation may lie in the set of values on which the Healthy Cities strategy is based. These are the beliefs that health is a legitimate area for public action; that health should be considered an essential human, social and physical resource; and that the aim of public health action should therefore be to create the conditions in which health can be developed and sustained. Values are identified as an important characteristic of health promotion practice by Downie and his collaborators (Downie *et al.* 1990). In order to assess the impact of Healthy Cities in Europe, it will be important to know how widely these values are accepted, by which social groups and whether they make a difference to health promotion practice.

Research on actions to improve health which are carried out within a Healthy Cities framework could profitably consider the relationship between the meanings given to health and the initiation of action to improve health or the environment. Definitions of health used in Healthy Cities include health as a 'community resource' and health as an 'active process created and lived by people' (Tsouros 1990b). Local actions undertaken under the umbrella of Healthy Cities projects often include the direct participation of lay people in defining the health needs of their community. In Nancy and Munich and the Healthy Schools approach developed by Horsens, the direct participation of children has encouraged action on health and environmental change. It will be important to explore the importance of associating a positive view of health with participative processes in empowering people to take action on health and environmental issues.

It has been argued that an assessment of the significance of Healthy Cities involves attention to the importance of symbols and perceptions, as well as of practical actions. The use of the concept of locality within Healthy Cities provides a useful focus for the convergence of research and health promotion interests. Within Healthy Cities the concept of locality is complex and variously applied. Associating health with the symbolic meaning of the city has had success in winning political commitment, but the political and administrative authorities associated with projects have not been confined to those at city level, and activities have often been more local (Curtice and McQueen 1990). These diverse interpretations of the city do not constitute a paradox when the city is viewed as an example of the functional and symbolic use of different settings in health promotion practice. The rationale for developing a health promotion agenda within particular types of setting such as the workplace, the city or the school, is that the place selected represents a social nexus and provides a common focus for associated groups; thus the strategy is twofold: to improve health within the setting and to raise awareness in coalitions built around the setting (Ilona Kickbusch, Planning meeting for the Healthy Schools Project, WHO/Euro, April 1991).

From a research perspective, it is the relationships between place, meanings, structures, social processes and actions created within a particular setting that are of greatest interest. One test of the Healthy Cities strategy will be how far the focus on the city/locality leads to renewed attention to the physical, cultural and social contexts of communities in relation to health. There are some suggestions, in the available material on models of good practice, that the processes involved in local health promoting activities are synergistic. For example, in projects which participants themselves identify as successful, intersectoral collaboration is seen as a way in which locally identified issues can become the focus for broadly based action in particular localities (preliminary analysis of 1990 Healthy Cities questionnaires).

Starting from the definition of health in Healthy Cities and Health for All, it may, therefore, be feasible to develop outcome criteria for project evaluation which are intelligible both in terms of health promotion practice and in social research on health, namely, the development of individual and group skills, increase in perceived control over the conditions which create health, the development of structures and processes to improve health conditions, an increase in health resources in the community and improvements to environmental conditions.

CITIES RESEARCH STRATEGY: AN IMAGINARY DEBATE

It is impossible to discuss the research implications of the experience of the first five years of the WHO Healthy Cities project in Europe without confronting the puzzle: why has research and evaluation apparently had such a low profile?

Lack of infrastructure for international research co-operation, particularly in the 'softer' sciences, has presented probably the most serious limitation on the development of co-ordinated and high-quality research responses during the first phase of the Healthy Cities project in Europe (Curtice 1991). The project has demonstrated the need for funding for the development of international research networks and for collaborative research projects. Such projects could investigate a core set of research questions in different settings and compatible and complementary methodologies could be compared between research teams. It must be acknowledged that the present lack of harmonization between the collection of much health-relevant data makes it difficult to address adequately the information needs of any international health project. The funding situation is, however, likely to improve during the lifetime of the second phase of the project as the European Communities have begun to adopt measures to create a 'researcher's Europe' with opportunities, not limited to the hard sciences, for collaboration between research centres (Newby et al. 1991). A research network to evaluate European health practice has now been funded by the European Community.

Resources will not be enough, however, if strategic, practical and academic interests do not find points of convergence. The present section reflects on the basis for exchange between practitioners and researchers within Healthy Cities networks. What resources might be exchanged, what strategies are most likely to lead to the development of programmes of shared interests, what are the obstacles to collaboration and what benefits might be obtained from it? The context and background for research involvement will be considered through the device of expressions of interest from some selected, but imaginary, interested parties, in order to highlight some of the issues implicitly at stake in approaches to Healthy Cities research.

There are several reasons for adopting the device of an imaginary debate to illustrate the opportunities and the difficulties of greater research involvement in Healthy Cities. In the first place, a debate between research perspectives is the preferred approach for the development of a Healthy Cities research strategy. A pluralist approach befits the many diversities within the project and the wide range of potential research interests which might be appropriate to its research needs. A simulated debate is also intended to highlight the need for a process, most probably on the model of coalition-building or networking, through which researchers could more effectively become involved in Healthy Cities. For such a process to get under way it would first be necessary to identify more clearly than hitherto the interests of all parties, including the research community, as a basis for co-operation. Yet in many ways, what follows is not so much a debate as a series of preliminary positions. These caricatures of various academic and public responses are intended to illustrate the point that there are currently varying levels of engagement with public health issues in different disciplines. Moreover, while there is work in many fields which is of great potential relevance to Healthy Cities policy development and evaluation, it is not automatic for these links to be perceived. Before multidisciplinary Healthy Cities research can develop, questions need to be formulated in a way which attracts the interests of different disciplines and, for their part, researchers need to take on board some of the concerns of the public health movement. Differences in research paradigm, methodological approach or political position may also affect research involvement. Most of all, however, an exercise in alternative history is reported because, as yet, there has been limited research engagement with Healthy Cities. Traditional solutions to Healthy Cities research problems are unlikely to prove satisfactory and it is therefore suggested that realignments within research and between researchers and practitioners may be called for. New partnerships are needed to build a coherent research response.

A debate

The public health physician's perspective:
My view as a public health doctor is that emphasis on the city is justified on demographic grounds. Health problems in post-industrial cities present as formidable a challenge to public health as the spread of infectious diseases in the last century. But public health action today needs to be underpinned by the development of a *social* epidemiology which is sensitive to the complex aetiology of contemporary health problems; to the interactions, for example, between occupational risk, stress and health behaviours (Anderson *et al.* 1988). Healthy Cities appears to confuse process and outcome. It is not clear to me how the action undertaken by these projects is expected to result in improvements to the health of specific population groups in European cities in, say, ten years' time. What specific health targets is the project aiming at and how does it intend to measure improvements in its chosen health indicators?

If you ask me what contribution the public health sciences could make to evaluation of the Healthy Cities project in Europe, I would say that they have a key role to play. The tool of community diagnosis has been developed to identify health needs at the local level (Bethell

1991; Sainsbury 1991). There is great technical expertise in the environmental health sciences in measuring pollution levels and in setting standards of environmental quality, for example air quality. The public health sciences are well placed to assemble baseline data on the health of city populations and to monitor changes in health indicators. There are now established approaches for measuring quality of life (Bowling 1991).

The public policy analyst's perspective:
Speaking as a public policy analyst, the main difficulty I have with what I have read about Healthy Cities so far is that the literature seems to spring out of nothing. I would like to see it analysed – to give an example – in terms of the broader debates about the effectiveness of public welfare programmes and the balance of state and voluntary action in the historical development of social welfare (Cawson 1982; Glazer 1988; De Swaan 1988).

The way you have outlined the project also seems to make insufficient allowance for the differences in the administrative structures within which health policies are formulated in the various European states. Is it really possible to generalize about the policy process in, for example, the Netherlands and Italy? I would suggest a set of national case-studies to show why particular health policy options get taken up, and which policy processes are favoured in particular institutional contexts (De Leeuw 1989a; Dekker and Saan 1990; Healey 1990).

The political scientist's perspective:
There seems to be an assumption in Healthy Cities that health is a consensual value. From a political science perspective, I see a contradiction between this assumption and the proposition that the Healthy Cities project is a vehicle for action on social inequalities (Byrne 1991). Within what framework of political theory is the project's advocacy of public participation being developed (Rifkin 1981)?

I would like to see analyses of which groups come to be represented through Healthy Cities projects, whose interests prevail, and how far the results of these processes are successfully translated into policies to promote equity. How successful is the project's penetration of urban elites (Judd and Parkinson 1990) and how is conflict resolved in the Healthy Cities process? (Baum 1990).

The sociologist's perspective:
I had never heard of Healthy Cities. It reminds me of sociological

debates we had in the sixties about the nature of communities and methods for community studies (Bell and Newby 1971).

In terms of bringing a sociological perspective to the problems which Healthy Cities is interested in, you would obviously want to build on the traditions of urban sociology and perhaps look at the health careers of different social groups in the city as aspects of the social relationships and expressive orders being played out within the various physical spaces of the city (Dickens 1990).

I am not sure, though, how far Healthy Cities has really put an ecological perspective into practice. The language of Healthy Cities is about social change, but I see no indication that health promotion has engaged meaningfully with debates in social theory (Beattie 1991).

I am sceptical about the claim that Healthy Cities is a social movement; it seems too closely tied to the interests of an international bureaucracy and various professional groups (Stevenson and Burke 1991). There is a gap between the rhetoric and the scale of action you are describing. I think my first question would be 'Does the emperor have any clothes?' You have to ask yourself whose interests are being served by the adoption of health and participation as a new form of political rhetoric (Strong 1986; McQueen 1989; Kelly 1990c).

The social geographer's perspective:
It would be interesting for social geographers to know about any specific projects Healthy Cities are undertaking to improve health through attention to the built environment. Housing policies, for example, can affect health through various routes and it would be valuable to explore more closely the relationship between these policies and their health impact (Smith 1989).

There is a difficulty in conceptualizing all urban health environments as similar. An example of a research subject which might make it possible to highlight the effects of historical and social context in different kinds of urban space is the health experience of women in cities (Mackenzie 1988).

The health promoter's perspective:
The Healthy Cities project is putting into action many of the tenets of health promotion. Research on the project is needed to provide concrete illustrations of the processes by which people at the local level can take an active role in creating positive health and to show the significance and feasibility of public policy action and organizational changes in improving health chances (De Leeuw *et al.* 1990).

As health promoters we would see the need for two levels of research input: applied research which will tell us which approaches are effective and worth implementing more widely, and policy analysis which will bring out the rationale and implications of strategic decisions. We would expect to see research practices developing which themselves make use of social learning theory and diffusions of innovations theory, and draw on the experience of major community-based health initiatives to integrate research and evaluation into the design of the programme and to disseminate the results of research rapidly back to practitioners in order to impact on future strategy development (Bracht 1990; Richardson *et al.* 1990; Tones *et al.* 1990; Crosswaite and Curtice 1991).

The community activist's perspective:
Community activists hope to influence the Healthy Cities project, to put into practice what it says about participation and about the need to prioritize the issues which local people think are important. We would therefore like to see research commissioned by the Healthy Cities project to look at the health issues which matter to people in those cities such as the health risk of environmental pollution, the effects of poverty on health and unequal access to services. We are not looking to the Healthy Cities project for answers, but we think that it has an important role in legitimizing community-based approaches to health. Research can provide useful ammunition in local campaigns, and we also think it could have an important strategic role in showing how local government policies need to be changed if action at the community level is to have any impact. Most academic research is too abstract to be of any use to the people on whom it is conducted. We would argue that practitioners and ordinary people could take a much more active role in carrying out Healthy Cities research, that research practices need to become more open and participative and that researchers should be made accountable to local people when they do research in communities.

The city politician's perspective:
When I first heard about Healthy Cities I thought it was stronger on diagnosing the problem than in providing solutions. Now that it has been up and running for a few years I expect the research to be able to tell me and politicians like me, whether the project has worked. I hope to see evidence that investment in social programmes can be justified in terms of improved health for our most vulnerable citizens and I need to know which are the most effective uses of limited resources. I want to be able to cite specific examples of the benefits of taking health impacts into account in transport, waste and planning policy.

These are some of the voices which we may imagine would assail the ears of a putative research development officer for Healthy Cities in Europe. What conclusions might she draw? She might be forgiven for being initially disheartened by the academic response; scepticism seems to be the order of the day. Then there are very few research responses which seek to engage with the whole of Healthy Cities; most identify a particular area where their empirical work most easily fits. On the other hand, the list of disciplines which seem to construe Healthy Cities as their territory is very long. How could these different research claims be prioritized? There is precious little here about how research could solve the pressing strategical and practical needs of the project for a better information base and for usable findings (Lawler *et al.* 1985).

There is a noticeable difference between the initial responses of the researchers, whose tendency is to engage critically with the concepts of the project, and the kind of research response which the practitioners, represented here by the health promoter, the community activist and the politician, expect. They engage critically all the time with the concepts and practice but what they want from research is a practical contribution which will take that debate one stage further. They need information urgently about how the concepts work in practice, and they want assessment of the effects of particular policy options. Research involvement is not, however, required at any price. Healthy Cities is developing a style of practice, and research should be sympathetic to that way of working.

CONCLUSIONS: ON RESEARCH DIRECTIONS WITHIN THE EUROPEAN PROJECT

This imaginary debate and reflection prompt some suggestions about the prospects for a realistic research agenda for Healthy Cities in Europe. The gap between the research needs of the project and the available research responses needs to be bridged through a process of active debate. There are presentational issues for the project to consider if it wants to stimulate research in particular areas. The implications of the overall project strategy may be more usefully approached by researchers through a pertinent issue from their own subject area. Multifaceted issues such as the health of women within the city would provide a focus for interdisciplinary discussion within which specific research questions could be debated and developed (Orr 1987). A thematic presentation of research areas, whether based on a population group, or an issue such as healthy transport, also provides a structure within which it is possible to consider international comparative work and, not least, to seek funding for it. Themes help to define the practitioners and researchers who might have an interest in the area. The particular philosophy and approaches associated with the project may be more meaningful when presented as a new synthesis within a particular field.

The use of themes is not, however, an alternative strategy to a focus on city or locality, as the selection and prioritization of themes would be done within each city. Existing issue-based working groups and the work plans for producing city health plans provide a framework for the development of research strategies. There is, however, no logical reason why the most appropriate research technologies should be based in the cities which identify particular problems. Hence, networks of cities, such as those established around the multi-city action plans, could be used as a way of developing and sharing research expertise. As in other areas of activity, Healthy Cities practitioners will find that there are other networks to which they will also have to relate, even though Healthy Cities interests are fairly marginal to those. It may be worth considering what Healthy Cities has to offer professional scientific networks; one answer lies in its established European links and existing coalitions of lay and technical staff.

Other problems highlighted by the imaginary research debate about Healthy Cities concerned differences in perceptions of the nature and significance of the project. The conclusion is inescapable that these differences should not be excluded from the research agenda but, rather, explored within it. The argument has been made that Healthy Cities is attempting to create the context for the implementation of Health for All strategies by altering the terms of the debate about health. Disagreements about the nature and origins of its ideology and the perceived significance of its thought and activity within different intellectual traditions therefore, have a legitimate place within this wider strategy which entails, not only the building of social and political coalitions, but also influencing the associations between concepts, the meanings of words and the recognition of symbols. Debates about legitimacy, relevance and significance can be conducted on equal terms between practitioners and researchers since both are concerned in them, and provide an avenue by which the project can participate in the formulation of the terms of reference by which it will be judged.

The logic of this argument leads to the conclusion that a Healthy Cities research strategy needs to refocus upstream in its engagement with intellectual debate. Otherwise, the possibilities for dialogue with ideas and practices in other related fields may never be fully realized. Moreover, the research agenda which is produced is unlikely to contribute much to the questions underlying key project objectives. For example, inter-agency work is one of the central processes recommended by the Healthy Cities strategy; it is valued as a mechanism for building coalitions in order to get health put on the policy agenda. The practice of inter-agency work is also recommended in other areas of practice within the human services, notably social welfare (Dluhy, 1990). A research question which could be examined within Healthy Cities and would then contribute to the assessment of inter-agency work in more than one field would be, does inter-agency work lead to greater policy responsiveness? Here is a question which requires theoretical, empirical and practical examination, the conclusions of which would be relevant to the evaluation of Healthy Cities strategies and practice (Delaney and Moran 1991).

A restricted definition of evaluation requirements may be an obstacle to the utilization of research within the project (Patton 1986). In the short term, the pressures to demonstrate accountability to funding agencies and political supporters appear to require a strictly instrumental use of research. A developmental project must claim to be innovative and show solid results in order to win political support and resources. Yet confining the task of the evaluation to identifying what is new and effective in the project may be counter-productive to research involvement. The argument has been rehearsed that a claim to be innovative is likely to produce a sceptical response from the research community. An over-emphasis on the need to demonstrate clear results from Healthy Cities intervention will favour the use of more established research technologies. Not only may reliance on these be inappropriate to the demands of the project, but it will reduce a major incentive for research co-operation, the possibility to develop and apply new methodologies.

There are some paradigms and methods for evaluation research in which the different interests of parties with a stake in the evaluation are clarified and the different meanings of success are openly addressed. In this view of the evaluation task, the clarification of goals with all the participants in an activity itself becomes a strategy for evaluation. The term 'pluralistic evaluation' has been used to describe the application of such an approach to the study of health care which involved measuring success according to various criteria which reflected the goals and values of different groups within the agency being studied, such as managers, professional staff, users and carers (Smith and Cantley 1985). The most radical development of a negotiated approach to the conduct of evaluative research has come from Guba and Lincoln who, in 'fourth generation evaluation', advocate an evaluation process which incorporates feedback between the providers and interpreters of information at every stage, including establishing the definitions of success (Guba and Lincoln 1989). This interactive and reflexive framework for evaluation seems potentially compatible with the participatory methods favoured in community health work practice and may, therefore, offer an important bridge between research conducted in and with communities to identify their health needs, and evaluation strategies to review the responses of agencies to new ways of working.

A research strategy is also one way to avoid an eclectic approach to research which rummages for the most appropriate technique for the occasion, only to be dismayed when it proves to be a tool for answering an entirely different kind of question. Research is not value free and techniques are usually not separable from their theoretical and philosophical basis (Research Unit in Health and Behavioural Change 1989). Health promotion practice, as exemplified by Healthy Cities, will be ill-served by an unselective approach to research which adopts the nearest method to hand. This is not a basis for co-operation between practitioners, researchers or communities. As an exponent of the use of qualitative research approaches in the evaluation of healthy public policy and practice, I sometimes feel myself, when at health promotion research meetings, to be manning a market stall – 'Buy my in-depth wares', I shout. A young community physician, charged with carrying out a community-based needs assessment, rushes eagerly to my stall, under his arm a sheaf of reports on community health profiles and ethnographic appraisal. Then other cries are heard: 'Environmental indicators, environmental indicators', 'cross-national risk scores, sweet risk scores' and off he goes to be beguiled by other research methods packaged for application to his needs. But if different research techniques are a shorthand for different philosophical positions and ways of responding to the world, what will be the consequences for the communities involved and the quality of the information produced, of this shopping about for usable research strategies? In Elizabethan times the musical art of the composers Gibbons and Weelkes was able to blend English street cries into the music of the famous *Cries of London*; it will take a concerted effort by practitioners and researchers to develop acceptable and effective ways of implementing a coherent Health for All research agenda. The development of that agenda requires a climate of open debate, a structure of collaborative networks and a process in which the meaning and methods of practice and research can be negotiated.

ACKNOWLEDGEMENTS

I am grateful to David McQueen, Ron Draper, the staff of the Healthy Cities Project Office and the Healthy Cities project team, for their ideas, experiences and enthusiasm. The opinions expressed, however, are those of the author.

The Research Unit in Health and Behavioural Change is funded by the Chief Scientist office of the Scottish Home and Health Department, the Health Education Board for Scotland (HEBS) and the Economic and Social Research Council (ESRC); however, the opinions expressed in this chapter are those of the author, not of the funding bodies.

Chapter 5

Walking the tightrope
Issues in evaluation and community participation for Health for All
Jan Smithies and Lee Adams

INTRODUCTION: PARTICIPATION AND HEALTH

This chapter has been prepared by health promotion practitioners with experience at local and national level who are concerned with involving people in activity to promote health and the Health for All movement. As part of their experience over a number of years, they found that there often appeared to be a lack of academic support in Britain for participatory approaches for the research and evaluation of health promotion and Health for All. This needs to be remedied in order to enrich and develop work in statutory organizations, and to be a resource to communities concerning their health. The chapter provides a rationale for the importance of research and evaluation to complement a participatory and community development philosophy and methodology. It seeks to describe levels of participation and the complexity of research questions and debates, to highlight some of the dilemmas inherent in working in this way, to describe case-studies illustrative of points in the chapter and to draw conclusions.

Researchers who are involved in community development and health need to work with the principles of Health for All and incorporate these into research processes. Such researchers face the task of 'walking the tightrope' between conflicting expectations, philosophies and demands – such as the immediacy of service delivery, the politics of health bureaucracies and a remote academic community (Baum 1988: 260). Baum suggests that the researcher must develop a good sense of balance! This chapter is an examination of some of the processes, tools and theories that are important in developing such a sense of balance.

In recent years, community participation has become a central tenet of health promotion. The International Conference on Primary Health Care held in Alma-Ata in 1978 emphasized community participation in health. The declaration stated, 'people have a right and a duty to participate individually and collectively in the planning and implementation of their health care' (WHO 1978: 20). In 1986, the 'Ottawa Charter' which developed the Alma-Ata principles stated, 'Health promotion works through effective community action in setting priorities, making decisions, planning strategies and implementing them to achieve better health, at the heart of this process is the empowerment of communities, and the ownership and control of their own endeavours and destiny' (WHO 1986). Community participation is integral to the WHO Health for All strategy which recognizes that it is only the involvement of people in health issues and the factors that affect health, that can bring about the changes necessary to reduce health inequality and promote well-being.

Closer to home, the British Government, in the National Health Service (NHS) reforms of the 1980s and early 1990s, emphasized that services needed to be more responsive to consumers' rights and that consumer involvement should be more than a 'rubber stamping' exercise to health authority decisions (DoH/NHS Management Executive 1990). Participation is, however, not just about rights, important though these are. Physical health benefits have also been demonstrated, in that participation can affect the body's defence system and decrease susceptibility to illness (Cohen and Syne 1985).

However, in extolling the virtues of participation it is naive to think that grass-roots work and some local state responsiveness will dramatically improve health. Reducing inequalities will require a redistribution of resources and power in society and political change at governmental level. Participation in health, enhanced by community development approaches, can exert an influence on the local state and create movements for change. This produces short-term material gains such as changes in the way health centres are run, and also the formation of anti-poverty and anti-discriminatory programmes, for example.

The community health movement in the UK (including the black health movement and women's health movement) which encompasses participatory approaches, has a vibrant history of twenty years or more (Adams *et al.* 1990). It comprises the community development approach within health projects and includes health and social welfare practitioners committed to developing innovative service provision. Evaluation has been undertaken in much of this work and recently a review was completed (HEA/OU 1990). There have also been some radical community-based research projects investigating how health needs are perceived by ordinary people. Some of these have been based on community development methods and involve the community at each stage of the project (Prout 1990).

Community participation is integral to the Health for All vision and strategy. It is a challenging agenda as it goes beyond consultation on already formulated plans to involvement of communities in the issues which affect health and well-being. Citizen community participation in decision-making about health and the conditions that predispose towards Health for All were identified as essential to deal with the health policy changes of the twenty-first century by the Second International Conference on Health Promotion held in Adelaide in 1988. The main features of such approaches are that work is usually with groups rather than specific individuals, focuses on disadvantaged and/or marginalized groups, takes a positive, holistic view of health and is based upon a social model which acknowledges the effects on health of the environment, income and social circumstances. Such work aims to increase self-confidence, self-esteem, knowledge and skills, thereby *empowering* individuals and communities and allowing them to define their own needs. The process of the work is considered as important and health-promoting as any outcomes. Equal opportunities are promoted and anti-discriminatory practices developed simultaneously.

As well as being potentially health-enhancing and important as part of a democratic process, community participation is important in terms of effectiveness. Decisions made by the people concerned are often better than those made for them by others. Skills learnt through participation can be extended to other aspects of people's lives, including their political awareness, and can be expressed in the wider community. The experience of participation can lead to a general increase in confidence (Lifman 1978).

LEVELS OF PARTICIPATION

Participation can be undertaken in many ways, to varying degrees and at various levels. It is becoming increasingly important to distinguish organization participation from community participation (Figure 5.1). Many people actively participate in community groups or voluntary organizations but have little or no desire to participate in statutory bodies and decision-making structures. If ordinary people participate at all, their involvement is often marginal. For example, Healthy Cities initiatives sometimes refer to having made progress, or more often, not having made progress in increasing community participation. What is usually meant by this is that people are participating in, or are in partnership with, statutory organizations. By distinguishing community participation from organizational participation, the need for organizations themselves to change and develop in order to be open to community involvement is highlighted. All participation, be it at organizational or community level, needs to be

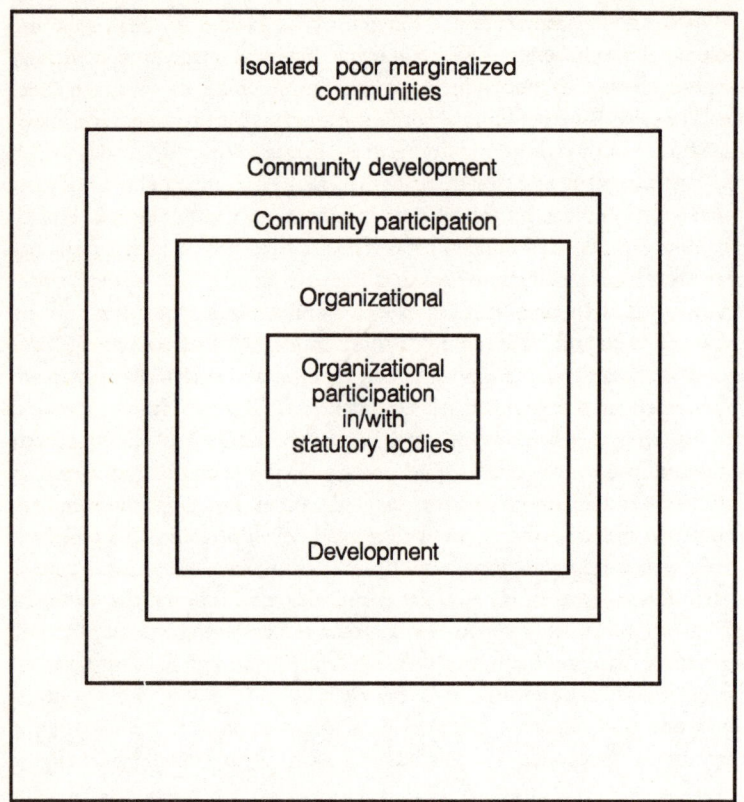

Figure 5.1 Levels of participation

stimulated by community development processes and practice if it is to be effective and meaningful.

Community development is a process whereby communities are empowered and enabled to express their health needs. People work on the ways these needs can be met collectively either through their own endeavours, at individual or community level, or through lobbying for action by local or national government or international organizations. Ideally, organizations have to be able and willing to respond to action stemming from community development, but also community development approaches can also involve conflict and direct action, to bring about change. To facilitate responsiveness and openness to community participation, a process of organizational development is required. Organizational development is an approach which can be seen to mirror the principles and methods of community development, but takes place within organizations at strategic levels. There is a great deal of management literature focusing on organizational development, but there has, as yet, been little work linking this to community development or participation (Smithies 1991).

Very few people in Britain take part in decision-making at organizational or formal levels regarding health and resource deployment. As health is largely defined with reference to illness, it is seen to be part and parcel of the NHS and placed in the hands of professionals or experts. But health is far more than the absence of disease, and many factors, most importantly social and economic ones, influence our health. We are all experts about our own health, and many different disciplines must be involved in improving health together with ordinary people themselves.

Even though few men and women are involved in decision-making within health services, everybody participates in their own health care and well-being and many people care for the health of others. Prevention requires a much more active role for lay people than curative services, which often require the client to be passive and compliant. Health Promotion requires active participants. This is a challenge for professionals who need to take on a different role in these circumstances and become partners in the process rather than experts. Organizations must expect challenges to the status quo.

COMMUNITY PARTICIPATION AND EVALUATION

Community participation strategies pose many difficulties for evaluation for a number of reasons. First, various actors and interests sometimes opposing each other may be involved; second, the work is developmental and outcomes are unpredictable; third, change takes place constantly; fourth, process is integral and needs evaluation as much as any outcomes; and finally, evaluation methods should mirror the principles of the approach itself. Evaluation of such approaches will assist in the development of understanding of individual, community and organizational development and behaviour in relation to health. What is needed is research and evaluation that focuses on illuminating the why and the how, as well as what and how many.

Community development has been described as a concept

> based on the premise that when people are given the opportunity to work out their own problems, they will find solutions that will have a more lasting effect. Hence... it is not necessarily the physical improve-

ments effected within a community, but principally the changes that have taken place in people themselves, that count as important in the process of community development.

(Anyanwu 1988)

This clearly has far-reaching implications for research and evaluation. Writers such as Anyanwu (1988) and Feurstein (1986) have promoted the concept of participatory evaluation as a method to fit the people, arguing that the use of such methodology means that both researcher and re-searched become partners in the joint venture of human liberation and mobilization (Anyanwu 1988). They and others have noted that problems of objectivity, validity and truth are often raised when qualitative research is seen to provide results which challenge the powers that be, and instead support the powerless and poor, challenging the notion that they should 'continue to be judged by others using sets of assumptions and value judgements constructed very largely without their participation' (Anyanwu 1988).

Many community health projects come up against the dilemmas ex-plored by Finch when outlining the relationship between research and policy. She notes that

quantitative researchers are not simply in the position of having to persuade policy-makers that their concept of 'objective' research is a naive one, but also have to cope with the reality that quantitative methods which provide 'objective research' are exceedingly useful in relation to the daily task of maintaining things as they are ... qualitative research, in contrast, is much more likely to offer up findings and insights which will disturb the status quo, while at the same time the methods employed make it impossible to claim credibility on the grounds of objectivity

(Finch 1986)

There is apparently a lack of political or scientific interest in advocating ordinary people's participation in research and evaluation. This, it has been argued, is rooted in an uncritical subservience to the mystiques of conven-tional evaluation approaches and an unswerving bias towards complex, costly and highly quantitative evaluation methods, resulting in an inability to perceive the need for a broader range of approaches, including particular skills that are needed to extend participatory principles to evaluation. It is suggested that the generation of large amounts of quantitative data becomes the private possession of a few, rather than being a resource for workers, participants and policy-makers involved in community development (Feurstein 1988).

These concerns are echoed in the Community Development and Health Project report of 1990. In exploring the background to a resource paper on planning, evaluation, research and accountability, it is argued that evaluation and accountability are more concerned with bureaucratic control than with allowing community health workers to develop opportunities for creative evaluation and action research. The report notes that these ideas were developed in response to the common experiences of frustrations and uncertainties in relation to planning, evaluation, action research and accountability in community health. The work is seen as an attempt to present an integrated account of these functions embedded within the theoretical framework of community development in health. However, the positive and creative methodology and theory explored and undertaken in their work is not often to be found within health promotion and Health for All research and evaluation.

Conventional evaluation methods are often held to be more objective, reliable and valid. This issue of validity is a crucial one when exploring participative approaches to evaluation. In such a process the researcher's or evaluator's role is not that of a producer of expert knowledge, but of a facilitator whose task is to support the development of the community's own knowledge. However, involving people in evaluating their own work, products and projects is often seen to introduce bias. There is a suggestion that people cannot distance themselves from their own participation sufficiently to make critical appraisals and evaluate what they have achieved and, most significantly, where they need to move forward to next. People active in the community health movement in the UK are only too well aware of how often their endeavour to take forward community development practice and principles into evaluation has led to criticisms of the validity of their methodology and data.

Brinberg and McGrath (1985) state that they wrote *Validity and the Research Process* as a reaction to the view of validity as something to be acquired by diligent application of certain techniques. They expand on this by arguing that

> Validity ... is a concept designated an ideal state – to be pursued but not to be attained ... validity is to do with truth, strength and value. The discourse of our field has often been in the tones that seem to imply that validity is a tangible 'resource', and that by applying appropriate techniques, one has somehow 'won' at the game called research.

However, claims of value-neutrality in policy research often run into conflict with principles of objectivity and practical demands for usefulness (Finch 1986).

Participatory evaluation is not a substitute for more traditional evaluation methods, rather it is a way to ensure that the approach and technology is more appropriate and effective and fits the needs of the people most closely involved in day-to-day community development work. Anyanwu (1988) is very clear about the importance of participatory evaluation:

> The process ... offers an educational experience which serves to determine community needs, as well as motivate citizens to develop the commitment to the solution of their problems. In this way, both the researcher and the researched become partners in the joint venture of human liberation and motivation.

Figure 5.2 illustrates the key stages in developing a participatory approach to evaluation. This is presented schematically, and it should be noted that many of the stages are complex and require a range of negotiation and facilitation skills in order to make progress in the face of lack of understanding or motivation from different interest groups. Training and development support may be needed throughout the process even at the initial stage in order to agree on a common understanding of the meaning and purpose of participatory evaluation (Step 1). The steps are presented as a circle to emphasize that the evaluation is a process, with each stage building up the basis for the next. Stage (11) is not an end, for participatory techniques are themselves a way of stimulating and initiating further community development action. The key skills needed by evaluators in this model include the ability to inspire confidence, to enable and facilitate skill development, and a commitment to empowering participants rather than holding on to 'expert' status. In effect the evaluator becomes a community development worker.

The steps in participatory evaluation are all developmental and have outcomes and implications far wider than just the evaluation itself. It has been argued that its meaning extends above and beyond seeing how much has been achieved or produced and at what cost and with what effect. The following outline, also derived from Feurstein (1986), illustrates this.

Participatory evaluation means:

- Building on what people already know and do
- Using and developing people's abilities and skills to monitor and evaluate their own progress
- Helping people to see whether their activities are having an impact on programme objectives

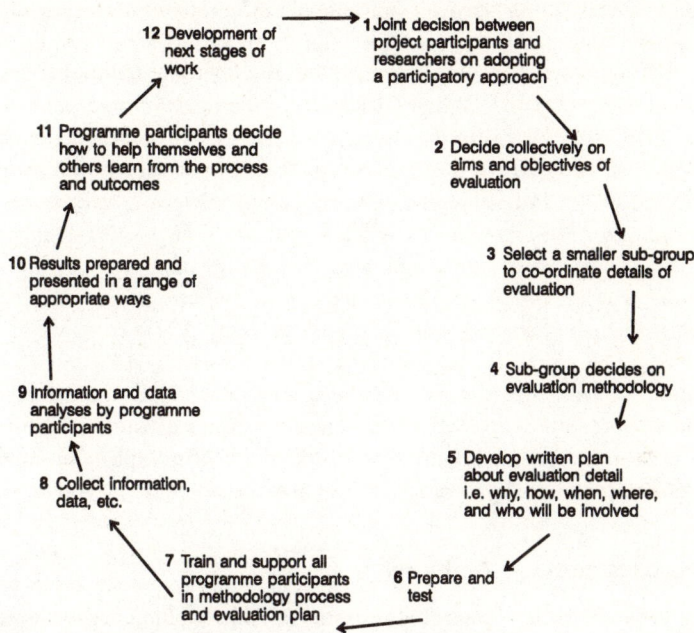

Figure 5.2 The participatory approach to evaluation
Source: After Feurstlin (1986)

- Revealing whether human and material resources are being used efficiently, effectively and at a cost which the programme can afford
- Enabling people to study their own methods of organization and management
- Providing good information for making decisions about planning and programme direction
- Indicating where more detailed information is needed and how it can be obtained
- Enabling people to see their own programme in a wider context, such as how it relates to other development work
- Enabling people to analyse their individual situations and to take action to improve them
- Increasing the sense of collective responsibility for programme activities

Despite the growing recognition that participative evaluation has a major contribution to make in reviewing and promoting Health for All work, it is fair to say that the methodology and principles are still anathema to most bureaucracies and institutions. As Jayne has noted, it has been left to 'small innovatory projects, such as community health projects, desperately trying to make their mark in a hostile economic and political environment, to develop evaluation theory and practice in this area of grass-roots development and provision...' (Inner City Health Project 1990).

Why have the majority of academics and social scientists working in health, social welfare and educational institutions not joined in partnership in this work and supported innovatory and liberating approaches to evaluation? The following case-studies are based on two national initiatives that the authors were involved with. In both instances they also include work that has a local grass-roots element. They illustrate attempts to put participative evaluation principles into practice. The first looks at the overall review and evaluation of the Health Education Authority's community development work, and the second concentrates on the Health Education Authority's 'Men Who Have Sex With Men – Action in the Community' project. Some of the difficulties help explain the unease academics and professional researchers may feel about involvement.

Health Education Authority

In 1988, the Health Education Authority (HEA) established a new division: Professional and Community Development (PCD). The authors of this chapter were appointed to the posts of Director and Assistant Director, Community Development, in the spring of that same year. The budget for community development work was initially very small, but soon built up to around £250,000 per annum. This was used to fund a range of strategic activities to support community development work from a national base. The overall aim was to build up an infrastructure that would both promote and support community development from the grass-roots level through organizational development at local and regional level to national policy-making. Thus, activities such as training, production of resources, supporting network development, and forums for information exchange such as workshops and conferences were financed. The work was undertaken in close co-operation with community health workers, projects and organizations. It was decided to mount an evaluation of the work of the division.

In determining both the style, methodology and choice of researchers for the HEA community development work, we were concerned to operate in a way that would increase skills, knowledge and conceptual thinking in this field. Thus, the use of methodology which reflected issues such as the importance of community participation, that was accessible and open to participants, and started from people's own perceptions of truth and reality was crucial.

A team was created composed of specifically selected individuals with practical experience in community development and health work as well as community development research and evaluation backgrounds. This was done in preference to establishing or using a traditional academic research department. The research and evaluation work was to be participatory, and therefore issues such as community development skills and experience, and a practice-based understanding of the importance of process as well as outcomes was central to the research methodology. It was felt that the credibility of both the researchers and their methodology within the twenty or so HEA-funded projects (each with their own workers and participant involvement) would be important in gaining access to the people's true feelings and perceptions about the change processes they were engaged in.

It is widely recognized and documented that community development workers have tended to view evaluation as a funder's tool, usually employing both personnel and methodology that are unsympathetic or inappropriate. Indeed, it sometimes seems to have been the case that the evaluation that was likely to be least sympathetic to community development was deployed and then produced results to justify closing down projects on the grounds that they were engaged in radical and political work.

Previously and until the work described here within the HEA, research was often of a highly quantitative nature and placed people and projects funded by the HEA in the position of subjects of research and evaluation, rather than active participants in the process.

It might be argued that staff engaged in research, like many other state-funded research organizations, function as technicians. Finch suggests that being cast in the technician role by definition gives the researcher a relatively limited amount of control over the kinds of data which are to be generated and the kind of issues which are to be studied (Finch 1986). It was our perception that the research departments of the HEA were used as the organization's gatekeeper to research knowledge and expertise; and struggles arose within the organization about who should make the decisions about research methodology and process. Those officials in the HEA with responsibility for community development (i.e. ourselves) began to suggest that a rather different approach might be needed to evaluate community development work.

The research task, as defined by community development work priorities and the Department of Health's review requirement, was to explore how effective community development was as a method of promoting health. A research brief about the nature and impact of the division's work was widened to include an exploration of the way that the HEA's own structures, policies and priorities aided or hindered the work of the Professional Community and Development Division.

The HEA and its predecessor, the Health Education Council, did not seem to regard the participation of its staff, procedures, culture and policies as relevant topics of research. Likewise, the wider context within which projects were expected to work (e.g. their connections to each other and their impact on the wider health promotion field, i.e. the strategic implications of work) was also seldom subjected to evaluation review.

The approach taken was to commission a qualitative piece of research involving a team of seven researchers over an initial three-month period. The team were co-ordinated by the Open University. Their preliminary brief was to map and review community development activities and strategies. This included process and policy as well as actual projects funded from the community development budget. The overall aim was to fund an in-depth research project for three years to evaluate the progress of community development, building on the initial review and analysis. This second stage was never implemented due to subsequent changes in the HEA's structuring and strategy with regard to community development.

The seven researchers all had discrete responsibilities within an overall team framework and aims. It was vital that the community development evaluation should base its analysis of the work in the context of both the HEA itself and the wider health promotion and community development and health fields. Clearly the activities of the Professional and Community Development Division (PCD) did not develop or operate in a vacuum and it was felt to be important that the team should look at the total strategy as well as at individual initiatives and the funded projects. It was felt that it was crucial to evaluate the work in the context of the HEA itself as an organization. As most of the HEA's community development work was of a national and strategic nature, it was also important to determine the impact of wider community development and health work funded by other agencies. As community development is fundamentally concerned with working against oppression and disadvantage, the evaluation team were asked to consider an equal opportunities and/or positive action perspective in all their work. Specific emphasis was placed on evaluating the work from a black and ethnic minority perspective as this was felt to be most in need of development and analysis within the HEA and within the community development approach. Figure 5.3 illustrates the range of perspectives that were brought into the initial review, and which would have been further developed had the full-three year evaluation been able to go ahead.

As well as engaging the active participation of people directly involved in funded community development initiatives, many people indirectly (or directly) affected by the work within the HEA itself and the wider community, for example women's and black health movements, were also contacted and involved in the initial research. The intention was always that the review outcomes should be fed back to all the people that participated in the review in order for them to have an input into both the next stage of the evaluation, and into decision-making about future work and funding priorities based on the findings and analysis. It was also hoped that the approach, the skills and expertise of the researchers, and the data itself could be more widely available to help support others in their own work, and to add to the development of theory and practice in community

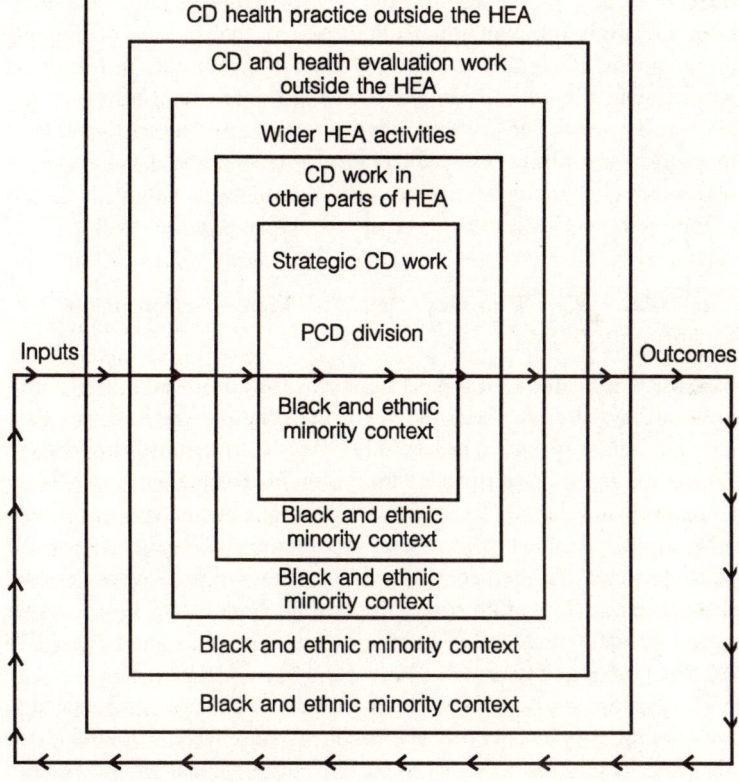

Figure 5.3 Evaluation perspectives

development and health work. The Open University (OU), who co-ordinated the research, submitted the initial three months' review of the HEA's community development work in the early spring of 1990; to date the document (over 200 pages of theory and practice data) remains unpublished.

The OU has continued a debate with the HEA about the need to publish, even if the HEA itself no longer considers the work appropriate or relevant. There are a number of reasons for this. First, the work is pioneering, both in terms of content and methodology, and is a much-needed resource for the community health movement in the UK and also internationally. Second, large numbers of people were interviewed by the research team, many of them working in community development and health projects completely unconnected to the HEA. They have yet to see the document. This is in direct contrast to the participative approach that they were initially involved in by the OU researchers. Third, reorganization effectively brought about the end of the HEA's community development strategy, and most of its funded community development projects, and the two senior community development workers left the HEA at that point. The OU review remains the only document, apart from internal documents, to record the rationale, process, and actual outcomes of community development work over the two-year period that community development operated at management level in the HEA.

MESMAC – Men Who Have Sex With Men – Action in the Community (HEA)

MESMAC is a three-year project funded by the Health Education Authority (HEA) within the HIV and Sexual Health programme; it began as a co-operation between this programme and the Community Development Division in the HEA at the same time as the work outlined above. It is a community development project working with gay men concerned with HIV and AIDS. The project is sited in four areas in England: Newcastle Social Services which works with men in urban and rural areas; Leicester Black HIV/AIDS Forum which focuses on black men; the Terrence Higgins Trust, working with young gay men in London; and Leeds AIDS Advice, working with gays in a large city.

The project is based on equal opportunities which are fundamental to the community development approach; gay men were involved in the planning, consultation, management and development of the project. Workers were encouraged by full and ongoing training and support to maximize community participation by basing actions on gay men's own needs. The particular interests of different communities of gays are respected and represented in planning, policy and decision-making and their life experience acknowledged as a form of expertise. Positive targeting is employed to ensure the involvement of under-represented groups such as black and ethnic minority men and disabled men.

Networking skills, knowledge and information-sharing are critical features of the approach. The project facilitators aim to empower gay men and enable choice and action on HIV/AIDS, at a personal, community, organizational and political level. The evaluation team based at Keele University are an integral part of the project and have developed close working relationships with project facilitators, project managers, the three project co-ordinators and the HEA staff. The evaluation draws on an approach usually called the 'illuminative paradigm' and utilizes Stake's concept of a description matrix (Stake 1967: 528). This seeks to provide a framework within which ongoing work and decisions can be monitored and reflected upon by all project members, and to provide an overall description and rigorous assessment of the project from which wider lessons can be drawn. The project requires not one evaluation but several, an overall assessment of aims and the study of several quite distinct local approaches. An attempt is made to produce a valid basis for comparison of local projects whilst remaining responsive to their unique contribution and situation. The study is caught in a number of tensions: a focus on outcomes as against an accurate description of process, between the need for a constant flow of formative feedback and the demands of a final summative assessment, and between expectations of participants within and without the project (Prout 1990: 15).

The design of the evaluation follows the principles of community development. Whilst rigorous and constructively critical, the evaluation acknowledges the importance of project members' own knowledge and insights and incorporates these into the overall evaluation picture. The evaluation also gives full feedback at all stages and levels of the project, rather than giving overall judgements at the end. In the case of MESMAC, descriptions of process and practices are vital; the identification, diffusion and application of good practice relies on knowledge of the how and why of practice as well as outcomes that were achieved. Evaluators in MESMAC are partners in the project and act as facilitators in the evaluation process. Thus all feel supported and enlightened by the evaluation process, and not intimidated or threatened. Evaluators in MESMAC and similar projects, therefore, need skills in negotiation, communication and relationship-building as well as research methodology.

CONCLUSIONS

The dominant evaluation paradigm in health promotion remains one which is defined as scientific, objective, neutral and providing a rational assessment of human performance. Practitioners of such evaluation are usually academics or professional researchers who work in education or research institutions. However, health promotion is complex and multi-faceted and draws on applied work of many different theoretical and practical activities. Mainstream evaluation objectives and methods are often inadequate and inefficient. This kind of work demands involvement with research subjects and action and development during the process of the research. It also means that research, action and evaluation need to be linked much more closely. They are still usually defined as different activities with different practitioners and skills. Evaluators need to be enablers, and the process of the evaluation itself needs to be actively useful to the people on whom the research is done rather than irrelevant or retrospective.

Evaluation and research within Health for All needs a radical rethink. It should employ the principles of the new public health movement:

- it should engage with participation as a dynamic in the process of the research and the way communities and the researched receive the research outcomes
- equal opportunities policies should be integrated into research methodologies
- researchers and evaluators should work in partnership with their subjects creating new methodologies
- researchers need to be accountable to their subjects
- the research process and intended outcomes should aim to contribute to reducing inequalities in health

The term academic needs to be redefined. Most workers in educational institutions have failed to embrace the Health for All movement; they need to be active partners, sharing their skills and resources and recognizing and legitimizing the important work being undertaken by the people for the people's health. Just as the community health movement has led the way in recent years in extending community development theory and practice, it should be possible for community participatory research in the health field to redefine methodologies and frameworks to create more liberating and illuminating ideas, knowledge and practice for the academic world. We need research for Health for All that is open and flexible and able to achieve an ethical balance.

Chapter 6

The relationship between research and policy
Translating knowledge into action
Sonja M. Hunt

INTRODUCTION: RESEARCH AND POLICY

The encouragement of more research and evaluation with respect to Health for All implies that research will somehow lead to action. That research might, or even should, be related to policy rests upon assumptions about both endeavours: that most research takes a form which makes it applicable to social problems and that policy is primarily influenced by evidence of a scientific nature. Arguably, both research and policy are influenced more by political expediency than by the desire for social justice.

The direction of most research in the public health arena is determined not so much by its social relevance as by its value to vested interests. Research becomes noteworthy less for its intellectual rigour, the excellence of its methods, the power of its results and the eloquence of its conclusions, than for its appeal to a particular ideological stance.

It is an illusion that there is a world where truth flourishes in the absence of power. Habermas (1971) believed that the very nature of science was such that it constituted a form of domination incompatible with humanistic and egalitarian pursuits, a belief echoed by others such as Bukharin and Virchow (Rosen 1979). Most research favours the privileged classes and they, in one form or another, largely determine the fate of the research. Members of underprivileged groups very rarely have any influence over either research or policy. It is scarcely surprising, then, that their interests are often overlooked in both arenas.

The notion that research can direct policy presumes that policy-makers work, at least some of the time, in such a way as to draw upon the most convincing and up-to-date evidence on any topic. Rather, however, it seems that social policy progresses less in a rational manner than by some form of muddle-headed incrementalism (Bulmer 1986). By and large, policy-makers seek to remedy current rather than future ills, many of which may be in-house rather than of significance to society at large, and work towards short-term rather than long-term goals. Decisions are rarely taken *because* of the evidence, rather evidence may be used to support existing positions and processes.

It has been suggested that, even where research has been deliberately initiated with policy decisions in mind, there is still little probability of the results being used. The normal life of academic research from inception to final report is three years, by which time the agenda for action will have changed, personnel will have moved on and interest in the topic is likely to have waned. Even where this is not the case, the results will still have to compete for time and debate with many other, mostly political, considerations (Weiss 1986). It has been said that, however relevant, important and well-argued at the proposal stage and however sound the results, research will have lost most of its appeal to the funders by the time a report appears (Thomas 1986).

Research may also be initiated as a way of not dealing with a problem as in 'We're awaiting the outcome of the research' or 'We're looking into it' or 'Our scientists are working on it right now', knowing that the issue will have died by the time the research is completed. In this way, researchers themselves can act as barriers to change by consenting to do certain kinds of work and by taking on work which will diffuse the issue either by 'technical fragmentation', that is, taking an issue out of its context, or by 'moral fragmentation', that is, treating people as objects, rather than speaking with them (Manning 1985). Generally, research strategies in public health fragment problems technically by addressing only a small part of a larger issue at any one time. Such is the case, for example, with smoking research. The medical model of human health encourages fragmentation by individualizing collective problems and researching accordingly, for instance by case finding, thus giving the impression that health problems are defined solely by medical diagnosis.

Researchers also act as barriers to change through their conservatism and career aspirations. Publication in an academic journal requires more than competence, it requires that the peer reviewers be pleased. Powerful academics can exert control over what is published, protecting and promulgating their own biases and vested interests. Publication tends to engender a sense of achievement in the researcher and a feeling that the task is done. Career advancement may depend upon being seen as 'sound' and not too controversial. Anecdotally, social scientists in particular seem more often than not to be socialist in their speech, but conservative in their behaviour.

The diversion of the issue of social inequalities in health away from social structure and living conditions into the field of lifestyles is a good example of some of these issues. Gusfield (1975) described the processes whereby groups who 'own' a problem, in the sense of having brought it into being in the first place, offload it by placing the responsibility for it onto other groups. Thus, explanations for the predominance of health problems in low income groups came to centre around individual behaviours such as smoking, alcohol abuse, poor diet and lack of exercise. As Weiner (1980) has described in relation to 'alcoholism', this involves a staged process of introducing the public to the idea, legitimating it by official recognition, showing it to be a big problem and then providing resources for investigation which academic departments and research units are keen to receive, often regardless of the intellectual dishonesty which is entailed.

This process allows control to be exerted over public facts, and the lack of funding for research on alternative explanations means that contradictory evidence is lacking (Farrant and Russell 1986). That the quality of the research is largely irrelevant to this process is well illustrated by work on heart disease and high fat diet, where all the 'best research', that is the most methodologically sound, has tended to show that there is no clear relationship (Kaplan 1988). The difference between a 'knowledge claim' and an acceptable fact, depends less upon the excellence of the research, and more upon the relevance of the material to ongoing pressures in the political arenas of local and national government and powerful cliques in the professional world.

Moreover, the bulk of research into public health matters describes, and does not explain, the issues examined. The research may thus raise a problem, but it does not specify what action is needed. If any action does ensue it will be firmly embedded in policy considerations.

The relationship between research and policy is thus complex. Knowledge is translated into action only under particular sets of circumstances, many of the elements of which may be entirely fortuitous.

CASE STUDY: RESEARCH ON HOUSING AND HEALTH

Background

From the beginning of the public health movement in the middle of the last century until the 1950s, it was widely accepted that housing conditions and ill health were closely linked and various public health reformers focused upon the provision of adequate dwellings as prerequisites for the prevention of health problems. The decline of tuberculosis after the Second World War seems to have led to an assumption that health hazards associated with housing had been eliminated. At the same time, there was a drive to build homes quickly to house people involved in slum clearance, as well as those who were victims of the gentrification of former working-class areas. People were often moved from their homes in the middle of town to peripheral areas, as happened in Glasgow and Edinburgh. The boom in cheap and inadequate building materials, together with the rising cost of land, resulted in low quality housing in some of the least desirable locations, for example, on low-lying, badly drained land exposed to prevailing winds. Whereas in the 1920s specifications for housing had often taken account of the health aspects of design, including adequate space and light, such considerations were forgotten or ignored in the 1960s.

Some research carried out between the 1960s and the 1980s had focused on damp housing and respiratory disease, but failed to make any impact. There were many reasons for this; the research was usually carried out by doctors and it was scarcely a fashionable topic in medical circles. The extent of the problem seemed quite limited possibly because the studies were based upon case-finding and tended to underestimate the size of the effects. Methodology was often poor with non-comparable samples and investigator bias. Such studies were, moreover, tucked away in esoteric journals and were certainly not accessible to the people who might have been most interested, that is, those who were living in damp houses.

In addition, health problems were seen largely as the province of medicine and the vast majority of doctors viewed housing as a political issue outside the realm of their responsibility. The problem of housing as a hazard to health suffered technical fragmentation by being split into separate domains. For example, the study of allergies as a consequence of contact with mould was largely the province of doctors interested in respiratory medicine; measuring dampness in dwellings was the province of environmental health officers; surveying and identifying mould in housing was confined to building researchers and microbiologists; investigating structural problems which gave rise to damp was the domain of architects.

Concurrently, moral fragmentation developed along two lines. The first was the promulgation of the idea that the ill health of individuals in bad housing was primarily a consequence of poverty and bad habits, and the second was that dampness in housing was also largely a consequence of individual behaviour such as breathing too heavily, boiling up nappies on the stove, making endless pans of mashed potatoes and taking baths!

The inhabitants of damp dwellings were largely disregarded in these investigations, useful only as objects of study, in spite of the fact that by virtue of their unfortunate situation, they could be regarded as participant observers on the topic of housing and health.

The first study

In 1983, a community development project was set up in a deprived area of Edinburgh. It was funded by the Scottish Home and Health Department and initiated by doctors concerned about the high levels of illness in the area. The idea was to get people to take more interest in health issues and, in particular, to persuade them to take up screening and give up smoking. However, the community worker who was appointed to the project held more participatory views, and local people were encouraged to define their own agenda for health.

A recurrent concern of tenants of the council was housing conditions, and in the summer of 1985, the Women's Health Group made a slide tape called 'Home, Sweet Home' which targeted the distress caused by damp and mouldy homes and the difficulties of persuading either the housing department or medical practitioners to take action. This tape was presented at a seminar at the University of Edinburgh and attracted interest, sympathy and praise. As the audience got up to leave, one of the tenants pointed out, rather angrily, that everyone thought it was a terrible shame, but nobody did anything.

Research is almost never initiated by lay people, unless they are in some relatively affluent charitable organization. Certainly there are few precedents for a research project to be launched by the 'disadvantaged'. The fact that this happened has to be attributed more to coincidence than to design, but as a consequence of the seminar, a small team of individuals from a research unit, community medicine, the community project, social workers and others got together to discuss the issue of housing and health and the possibility of carrying out a research project. Discussions were held with tenants about what form the research should take. Early on, two academics dropped out because they considered the issue to be too political, others dropped out because they thought the discussion too academic!

Eventually, a double-blind study involving 300 dwellings belonging to the council was carried out, whereby a face-to-face health survey was conducted first and the tenant asked to agree to a visit from an environmental health officer. A conditions survey of the dwelling was then carried out with particular reference to the presence of damp and visible mould growth.

The main findings are available elsewhere (Hunt *et al*. 1986a; Hunt *et al.* 1987; Martin *et al.* 1987). The important points to emerge were that the presence of damp was largely confined to certain streets and was related to the structure of the buildings, making it virtually impossible to attribute dampness to individual behaviour. There were strong and statistically significant links between the presence of damp and emotional distress in women and reports of respiratory, gastro-intestinal problems and infections in children. These results were independent of smoking, income, unemployment and other relevant variables.

The results were disseminated to the tenants' group involved, and public meetings were held at which members of the research team spoke. There were articles in the *Scotsman* and the *Evening News* and a television programme was made for Channel 4. The researchers went to considerable lengths to publicize the findings, but there was little local excitement, the original tenants' group had broken up and the issue was not pursued by the community project. A public meeting in the area where the research had been carried out attracted only eight people, of whom only two actually lived in the area. Another meeting, to which the eighteen general practitioners serving the target community had been invited to discuss an agenda for action with tenants, was attended by only one GP.

A paper sent to the *British Medical Journal* was rejected, apparently because the reviewer objected to the lack of association between parental smoking and children's respiratory symptoms. The authors protested at the tendentious nature of the review and wrote a rebuttal to the editor, whereupon the paper was sent to a different reviewer and subsequently accepted for publication.

The second study

Although the first study attracted a certain amount of interest and media attention, it certainly did not form the basis for any positive action on housing. However, the research team was keen to do a follow-up study and Glasgow District Council expressed interest in funding further work if the costs could be shared. The Glasgow Community Health Resource Unit was working with tenants interested in doing similar research in their area and they added weight to the proposal, as well as offering to assist in the research. Eventually, funding was promised by Glasgow and Edinburgh Housing Departments and the London Research Centre to carry out a study in the three cities.

Meanwhile, relationships were being established with the various tenants whose co-operation in the research was sought. It proved necessary to convince many people that the research was indeed for them, and not for the researchers alone. A potential barrier here was the popularity of deprived areas with those who did not live in them. Academics from various disciplines are notorious for coming to ask questions and then disappearing, with no discernible benefit accruing to the residents. Several stormy meetings took place which showed the bitterness and disillusionment with which many people regarded researchers who took all and gave nothing. In addition, the fact that the research was being funded by district council housing departments raised suspicions that a whitewash was planned. Eventually, mutual goodwill was established.

The research project was planned to have three parts:

1 A survey of the health of children and one parent in each dwelling;
2 A technical survey of the dwellings which would encompass structural features as well as the level of damp and mould and would include sampling of fungal spores in the air;
3 Analyses of mould taken from the dwellings

The plan thus rested upon the co-operation and co-ordination of many people of different backgrounds and different skills. Throughout, there was a great deal of co-operation and interaction between local officials, local people, the researchers and other agencies. This reached a peak in Glasgow where the tenants' groups were strongest and best organized. Among those collaborating in the study were:

– Officials of the housing departments concerned who provided addresses of tenanted properties
– Tenants and community councils who helped in identifying families with children and publicized the surveys, encouraging people to co-operate in a 'health survey' (An important task here was explaining why it was important that the purpose of the research was not explained at this stage)
– The Technical Services Agency in Glasgow – a tenant-managed architectural company who gave technical advice, recruited surveyors, and made space available
– Community workers who helped tenants to organize and provide space for meetings and discussions
– Members of the Department of Microbiology at Strathclyde University who recruited the microbiologist and provided laboratory facilities
– A member of the Environmental Health Department at Strathclyde University who worked out a system for classifying levels of damp and mould

- The researchers who were responsible for design, administration and co-ordination, analysis and dissemination of findings

The study was the largest of its kind ever carried out in Britain and established that there were dose–response relationships between the levels of mould in the air and on the walls and the extent and type of symptoms in children and that these findings were independent of smoking in the household, unemployment, income, household composition, the presence of pets and type of cooking facilities. They could not be accounted for by respondent, investigator or selection bias (Hunt *et al.* 1989; Hunt and Lewis 1989; Platt *et al.* 1989; Hunt 1990a).

The tenants were handed copies of the report as soon as it was available, at roughly the same time as the funding bodies received their copies. The researchers met with tenants to explain the significance of the results and to train them in the meaning of various terms. Workers in community education were also involved in helping local people with communication skills. The tenants set up press conferences in Glasgow and London, which they timed to coincide with the publication of the findings in the *British Medical Journal*. Questions were asked in the Houses of Parliament and the study appeared in parliamentary reports. The researchers gave talks to various community groups, to medical practitioners, to housing officials, to councillors and at national and international conferences. Interviews were given to the press and radio and both researchers and tenants appeared in a TV documentary. Numerous accounts of the research were prepared suitable for many different types of publications from community newspapers, to housing and public health journals, local government publications and magazines concerned with child care.

The housing department in Glasgow used the research to change its priorities in respect of renovations and to bring pressure to bear on the Government to allow more revenue to be raised for housing. Inside the council chambers the research created argument, provided a stimulus to action, raised the issue of housing higher up the agenda and led directly to a policy shift (Brooke 1990). For the first time the council publicly embraced the responsibility for ill health caused by its own housing and there were signs that tenants and council might make common cause. The Institute of Environmental Health Officers recommended a change in the 'tolerable standard' of dampness in housing regulations.

The research findings also influenced the obtaining of a grant by the Easthall tenants' group in Glasgow from the European Community for a £1.3 million Solar Energy Demonstration Project in Glasgow. The same group wrote and performed a play *Dampbusters*, which centred around the research. This play has been hugely successful and has been performed in front of many audiences throughout Glasgow and elsewhere.

The Right to Warmth campaign was set up, the aim of which is to work for warm, dry homes for everyone and the author became the convener of the health forum section of the campaign. The forum has recently produced a booklet entitled 'Unhealthy Homes' for distribution throughout Scotland to inform lay people of the health hazards of cold, damp and mouldy housing.

Some of the repercussions were, however, less predictable and less positive. Officials at the Scottish Office indicated their displeasure that the research had been done at all, that they had not been made aware of it and at the political implications. Warnings about career consequences, veiled and not so veiled, were received by members of the research team. A few members of more traditional Community Medicine Public Health departments showed signs of resentment that their territory was being poached upon by people who were not even medically qualified.

Jealousy and friction was also evident between tenants' groups as some appeared to get more publicity and more attention than others, and there was a feeling that some areas which were more visible in the media would get a disproportionate amount of housing money. The researchers were also treated with resentment by some community workers for pre-empting their role with tenants and for 'hogging' the publicity. There were also unforeseen medico-legal consequences. The research led to an increase in the number of tenants who brought legal action against Glasgow district council and the council found itself in the position of being sued on the basis of work it had itself commissioned.

Translating knowledge into action

This particular piece of research was unusually successful in triggering several types of action. The question is, why?

First, the research was grounded in an issue already of great importance to different groups. It was not, therefore, a case of researchers 'inventing' yet another problem. Damp housing has been a major concern in Scotland for a long time and has been thoroughly politicized. The public needed little convincing of its significance. As one of the tenants remarked, the results of the research 'showed what we knew all along'. In other words, the research was welcomed because it provided a 'respectable' and 'scientific' banner which could be waved by people already committed to the cause.

The findings gave heart to people, and the research was put into service of a position which had been reached on grounds other than those of empirical evidence, that is, social justice. Unlike much of the previous work on inequalities in health, such as the effects of low incomes and unemployment, the research involved the subjects in a meaningful way and was done primarily for them and shared with them, rather than invading their space and leaving them with nothing.

Second, tenants had been campaigning on the topic for many years, were committed to action and had access to various lobbies. They were unlikely to lose interest in a problem which had been afflicting them and their children for a long time.

Third, the study was not fragmented, either technically or morally, but adopted, as far as was compatible with good practice, a holistic orientation and approached the topic as a problem in community, rather than individual health. The research itself was scientifically sound, credible and explanatory, rather than descriptive, examining the causes of dampness and mould as well as the aetiology of symptoms. There were, thus, clear targets for action. The findings were capable of generalization and fitted in with a house conditions survey being compiled on all Glasgow housing. The size of the problem, the number of children who could be suffering was, therefore, able to be estimated and this added great emotional appeal.

The study had been funded primarily by district councils who had a vested interest in the findings for political reasons, and it gave them a lever for negotiation with the Government at a time when money for housing was being squeezed. The findings also meshed with other issues which were currently in the news: social inequalities, child poverty, use of energy/fuel poverty and the cost to health services. The involvement of the researchers after the completion of the study meant that it was hard for critics to distort the findings, oversimplify or dismiss them. The commitment of the researchers to proselytizing and to supporting the tenants' cause meant that a powerful alliance was formed between members of the public and the professionals concerned. The tenants could not be accused of exaggerating, fabricating or creating the conditions of which they had complained for so long. Equally, the academics could not be accused of being out of touch with the realities of public or private life.

The wide intersectoral collaboration ensured that there were several groups involved, each of which had its own network, facilitating dissemination of the information in diverse populations. Powerful allies already existed among members of the public, policy-makers and the media.

The research was also consonant with the new public health movement and thus acceptable by the radical community health set, as well as to more conservative and traditional researchers. (Although the research was methodologically sound, it should be recognized that the quality of the work was probably the factor of least relevance to its ability to provoke action. 'Bad' science can also flourish, especially when it is heavily supported by the establishment, is normative, and fits with political expediency).

Finally, and of crucial importance, the research was completed very quickly. The study began in January and the first report was ready by May of the same year. Thus, those who had provided funding and those who had supported the research in other ways did not have time to lose heart or to shift their attention to other issues. Once the results were made public, co-operation between researchers and tenants ensured that it was not a nine-days' wonder and even now, several years after the completion of the work, the consequences are still being felt and the alliance still exists.

CONCLUSIONS

The accumulation of 'facts' by means of the scientific method, as currently conceived, is an act of faith like any other and presents pictures of the world which are highly circumscribed in very particular ways. Research based upon 'science' is no more devoid of belief than policy based upon 'common sense'. There are many routes to knowledge, of which research represents but one, and one used by a minority at that. Government by scientists would be more sterile and uncomfortable than government by some form of democratic process, however imperfect.

Nevertheless, there are times when the brandishing of reliable and well-founded information can affect people's lives for the better. The public are relatively ignorant about the causes and prevention of ill health, by reason of their dependence upon gatekeepers who may, like the medical profession, have professional biases; like the politicians, have their own hidden agendas; like the media, be strongly influenced by both the former groups and the desire for a good story. Thus a gap appears between knowledge and public facts. Knowledge is relatively inaccessible to the public, but academics and researchers in the domain of public health are usually well versed in the conflicting findings of studies and competing aetiological models. They are, therefore, in the best possible position to convey the current state of knowledge (or ignorance) on a particular topic to the public.

There are, however, few incentives for academics to share their knowledge with the public or to assist in the promotion (or discouragement) of action associated with that knowledge. They will get no credit for it and it might harm their career. It will certainly take up time which could be spent writing more papers or attending conferences in exotic settings, even sitting on academic committees – activities which carry more weight on the scales of promotion than sitting in smoky halls talking with community action groups.

There is another health divide in addition to that between the social classes; this is the chasm between those who suffer from some social disadvantage and those who study it. A great number of academics have built reputations from work on social inequalities of various kinds, while those upon whom the work depended have benefited little, if at all, from the results. Using research to promote action requires that the researchers care as much about tackling the problem as they do about studying it and care enough to pool their knowledge with that of members of the public and policy-makers, instead of encasing it in an academic cocoon.

Research into health is a political activity by virtue of the availability of funding, the choice of topic and method and the dissemination of findings. There is nothing to be ashamed of in taking a moral stance and perhaps helping to redress social inequalities instead of contributing to them. An alliance between members of the public and academic or other researchers is potentially very powerful as it merges two disparate, but mutually enlightening, spheres of experience which can exert concerted pressure on policy-makers from two different directions at once.

Knowledge is more likely to be translated into action where there is a commitment by all concerned that this should happen and a willingness to work towards that end; where research is founded on the perceived needs of the public and put at the service of action groups who can utilize the information; where there is some political support for change; where it is clear what forms that change should take; where effort is put into maintaining interest and the pressure for action is sustained.

Above all, it is necessary that those involved respect and understand both the extent and the limits of their own expertise and that of the others.

Chapter 7

The ownership of research

Margaret Whitehead

INTRODUCTION

This chapter considers the control and manipulation of research and the power over knowledge that goes with it. The control over research exercised by various agencies and the consequences of that control for research in the healthy city is a key problem in bridging the gap between the aims and intentions of the Healthy Cities movement and its practice. In this context, ownership is a particularly significant force at the beginning and end of the research process. Before a project is initiated, ownership governs which topics are chosen for investigation and, to a certain extent, the methods employed. Just as importantly, it governs which topics are neglected or ignored altogether. Once research has been completed, ownership influences what is done with the results. It determines how, when and if, and for whose benefit the findings are disseminated. It is important to understand these issues of control and power in a community setting if ways are to be found of redressing the imbalance between the funders, users and practitioners of research and the communities being studied.

WHO'S IN CONTROL?

There are several potential stakeholders, or owners, in community health research, encompassing at least four broad categories, including:

1 the community in which the research takes place
2 the general public in whose name public funds are used and who may benefit from the results of research carried out on different sections of the population
3 professional research workers undertaking the investigations

4 the funders of the project and their associated policy-makers and politicians

In an ideal world, and in line with the Health for All strategy, the first category – the community – would figure as a central stakeholder. Priorities for research would spring from those identified by the community itself, based on that community's own particular needs. Moreover, people at every level would be involved in the choice of topics for research and the design and implementation of the research study. The widest possible participation at every stage would be encouraged. Likewise, the general public would have a strong voice in research decisions.

If the rhetoric is repeated often enough, some people, professionals and policy-makers alike, come to believe that this process is actually taking place on a substantial scale. But is it? What about the experience of this Swedish factory worker, commenting on an occupational health study? :

> Research seems often to be carried out above our heads. A couple of years ago I answered a questionnaire – it was sent out from the University. Some social scientists wanted to know about our working conditions and our views on different matters like work organisation – I don't remember everything. We have not seen or heard anything since. We don't know what they came up with. We have not seen any report – some of the questions were silly really. Do ordinary people like us have any possibility to influence the production of knowledge or is it only up to the researchers? If it is so, science is not very democratic in itself.
>
> (Starrin and Lundberg 1990).

This kind of experience and associated feelings of frustration are widespread and can be found in community health initiatives across Europe. Many communities find themselves powerless over the research activity taking place in their midst.

Neither are the professional researchers necessarily in as strong a position in terms of initiating research as perhaps they themselves would like to believe, though they do have more control than the communities they study. The rhetoric of the academic world perpetuates the image of the objective scientist, choosing a field of study, identifying problems for investigation within their special expertise, designing studies to elicit answers to the questions arising and carrying them out without contamination from outside influences, either from the object of the research or from political interference impinging from above.

Is this any closer to reality than the rhetoric of community ownership of research? Both the objectivity and freedom from outside influence are debatable. Indeed, there is growing recognition that no science is completely objective. Each person brings to their work their own particular view of the world, which influences them in the way they go about the research and in the choice of issues they see as relevant and suitable for study. This realization should not degrade the quality of research work as long as there is a recognition of the situation (Kelly 1990a).

Even when they have selected an interesting problem for investigation, many research workers will only go ahead and do the research if it is in line with the policy and priorities of the funding agency. Otherwise their projects would not stand a chance of obtaining funding.

The real power then, to set the research agenda, lies with the fourth category of stakeholder: the funders and their policy-making and political steering groups. In most community health research, the influence of the funding agency on the topics chosen for investigation is much greater than that of either the community or the research workers themselves. As many funders are health-related – the Medical Research Council, the Department of Health, the Health Education bodies (nationally) and regional and district health authorities (more locally) – a medical model tends to prevail. This has a built-in bias towards physical health problems, with the neglect of social and mental health issues. There is also a tendency to favour individualistic approaches, concentrating on investigations of personal behaviour in relation to health, at the expense of socio-economic and environmental factors. Overall, the top–down approach, with experts and official bodies identifying the research problems, tends to be dominant.

This can be seen at both the national and local levels where researchers may claim to be using community development techniques, but frequently the agenda has already been set by a health authority. In such cases, problems of low birth weight, low uptake of preventive services, high rates of coronary heart disease and lung cancer, will have been noted in certain deprived communities and the focus of the project is expected to be on those epidemiologically defined topics. No reference is made to the priorities of the residents of the communities on which the proposed projects are focused, and this goes against the basic principles of community development.

A glance at government-funded research and development in Britain reveals a preoccupation with current government policy initiatives in the process of being introduced (Cabinet Office 1990). For instance, priority areas for new research funded by the Department of Health are defined as:

- community care
- the acute sector
- workforce and personnel issues
- child care
- public health
- AIDS
- primary health care

Additional funds are allocated for research programmes on NHS equipment and supplies and NHS information technology.

On the one hand, these categories are so general as to be almost meaningless. On the other hand, closer inspection of plans indicates a preoccupation with narrowly defined health service issues, without the broad vision encompassed by the Health for All strategy. The Department of Health, it seems, is not interested in funding research on housing and health, transport or employment policies relevant to the wider public health. In recent years, there has also been a shift away from long-term research programmes towards funding short-term projects with the potential to deliver rapid results (Mays 1990). This system works against community development which is precisely the kind of process that requires more, not less, time to get established in the community and to bear fruit.

WILL THE FINDINGS SEE THE LIGHT OF DAY?

Researchers and their funders also have power over the findings of research studies. They control if and when the results will see the light of day, and to what purpose they are put. And anecdotally, there are many obstacles in the way of getting that knowledge to the people who form the basis of the research or to the public in general.

Researchers themselves create obstacles. Some take years to get round to analysing and publishing results, long after the time has passed when the results would be of use in policy-making. Others publish fast and furiously in furtherance of their own careers. However, because they have that particular aim in sight, they publish almost exclusively in academic journals and at conferences in a form and language accessible to only a few. This effectively excludes all but the most stout-hearted from discovering and understanding the research. Such researchers seldom see a responsibility for disseminating their findings to a wider audience of policy-makers and lay people in the community in which the study took place.

Still others, often unintentionally, are hoarders of precious information.

They use the research results to feed into and refine their next project. A typed report on the project goes to their supervisors and the funding body, and thereafter the report gathers dust on their office shelf. They explain, quite plausibly, that they are frantically busy, rushing from one project to the next, and simply have no time to stop and write up the results for a wider audience. Years later, they may contemplate doing something with the report but by then the information is too old. This neglect means that there is an enormous amount of useful, fascinating material languishing unpublished and therefore inaccessible to fellow researchers and the general public alike. It also leads to a great deal of reinventing the wheel, as successive researchers, who could have learnt from the experience gained in similar investigations, go on to cover the same ground and repeat the same mistakes.

The power to withhold useful research results is also vested in the funding bodies. Even when researchers are keen to disseminate their findings, their efforts, it has been argued, may be thwarted on occasions (Delamothe 1989). Information from research can be manipulated in a number of ways:

1 Publication can be held up for months or even years as completed research is passed from one official or committee to the next for approval. Further studies may be requested before the first results can be released. Commissioning further investigations or a working party to review the evidence can lead to years of delay. In this context, concern has been expressed about the possible effect of the new Department of Health (DoH) contract which all researchers now have to sign to receive DoH funds. This states: 'any publication of research material is subject to the prior consent of the Secretary of State which consent shall not be unreasonably withheld.' Some fear that this will lead to extra vetting and unnecessary delay of politically sensitive results. The department, for its part, has replied with reassurances that the contract will not be used for this purpose. The Association of Department of Health/Department of Social Security Research Workers, formed because of concern about the new contract, will be monitoring the situation and its effects on the principle of academic freedom (Zander et al. 1989).

2 Completed research reports can sometimes join mysterious publishing queues. There seems to be some law of nature that reports containing unpalatable findings get to the head of the queue and are published only when they are least likely to attract attention. In Britain, the Friday before a Bank Holiday Monday, especially in July and August when

half the country is on holiday, is a favourite time. This happened to the Registrar General's Decennial Supplement in 1986 (OPCS 1986) for example. Produced only once every ten years, it reached the front of the queue in August, four days after the House of Commons rose for its summer recess.

3 With more active news management, results can be released at the same time as a major new item. Royal weddings and outbreaks of war form very convenient smokescreens. If no major events are in the offing, then counter-events can be invented and staged to soak up the available space in the media.

4 Another ploy is to publish findings, but in an inaccessible form, difficult to get hold of. The 'Black Report' (DHSS 1980) is perhaps the best-known example of this, with just 250 copies of the 400–page document released in typescript form. For good measure it was published on the Friday before an August Bank Holiday.

These techniques can, of course, backfire. The medical press did not approve of the way the 'Black Report' was treated and gave it wide coverage. Similarly, when the update of the 'Black Report' – *The Health Divide* (Whitehead 1988) – was launched, cancellation of a planned press conference for the report led to widespread speculation about suppression of information and massive media coverage ensued. This ensured dissemination of the findings from local to international level, on a scale difficult to achieve intentionally.

POINTERS FOR THE HEALTHY CITY

With these very real problems and obstacles in mind, what lessons can be gleaned for the healthy city and its evaluation?

First, there are the problems associated with initiating research by a top–down process. Some of the power and control over what is investigated will only shift to the inhabitants of cities if researchers are more willing to share their skills and develop channels for bottom–up communication. There are examples of good practice in this field, including the collaboration between researchers and residents in Edinburgh on the subject of damp housing and health (Hunt 1987, 1990b), and the participatory research taking place between researchers and trade unions in Varmland in Sweden, to reduce health hazards in the workplace (Lundberg and Starrin 1990). There is much to be learnt from these initiatives, including the pitfalls to be avoided, as in the Italian experience (Reich and Goldman 1984).

A shift in power also requires recognition of the problem by funding bodies. Some will have been unaware of just how restricted their funding policy has been, and may be willing to broaden their approach once they understand the full picture. This is not a plea for all top–down research to be scrapped. Rather, it is an argument for complementary initiatives based on locally identified needs, covering social and environmental issues when they arise. There is also a need for more use to be made of sensitive qualitative methods of evaluation to enhance the quantitative approaches which have dominated the area so far. Such approaches are beginning to be explored and developed in the context of deprived city populations (Holman 1987; Hunt 1987).

Second, there are the problems associated with control over research results, and the lack of adequate dissemination. Researchers need to be encouraged to accept that an integral part of any study is the responsibility to disseminate findings as widely as possible and as quickly as possible. It has to be stressed more forcefully that researchers are falling down on their professional duty if they fail to make their findings accessible in this way. The obligation to disseminate does not stop at the door of the academic journal.

Again, there are examples of good practice. For instance, an integral part of the research and evaluation programme for Heartbeat Wales is the commitment to processing survey results rapidly and to produce reports that are widely circulated to policy-makers and the media. An outreach approach is employed by taking the results on a roadshow around the country, highlighting information of particular relevance to each locality.

With funding bodies, it needs to be stressed that an evaluation is incomplete without a dissemination phase. Moreover, that phase needs to feature in the overall research design right from the beginning and be suitably resourced.

Such moves by researchers and funders go hand in hand with initiatives to help people living in communities to gain access to the information they need, and to participate in research which will benefit them. These changes could begin to bring about a gradual shift in power, but there is also the need to be vigilant about the withholding of important information derived from research. The saying 'knowledge is power' is as relevant today as it ever was.

Chapter 8

Noarlunga Healthy Cities Pilot Project

The contribution of research and evaluation

Frances Baum

INTRODUCTION

The Noarlunga Healthy Cities Pilot Project was part of an Australian programme which sought to determine the applicability of the World Health Organization's Healthy Cities project to Australia. Noarlunga Healthy Cities evolved in a context in which significant community-based research work occurred both before and after the beginning of the project. This makes the Noarlunga experience a particularly interesting case-study of the ways in which applied research can support and contribute to a Healthy Cities initiative. The Australian Healthy Cities project and the local context in which the Noarlunga project developed will first be described and then the details of the research discussed.

HEALTHY CITIES AUSTRALIA PILOT PROJECT

Under the auspices of the Australian Community Health Association (ACHA), three Australian cities (Canberra, Australian Capital Territory; Illawarra, New South Wales; and Noarlunga, South Australia) were successful in applying for funding from the then (1987) Commonwealth Department of Health. The funding provided for a three-year pilot project by providing a national secretariat (co-located with the ACHA in Sydney) and a project staff of 1.5 in each of the three pilot cities. Co-ordination between the national secretariat and pilot cities was maintained by regular workshops, telephone conferencing and the routine exchange of project materials. In February 1989, these pilot cities were joined by a fourth, the Nganampa Health Council, which provides health services for the Aboriginal people living on the Pitjantjatjara lands in central Australia.

The national project was successful in attracting further communities to express interest in the Healthy Cities project. The national conference held in 1990 attracted 250 people. At the final session, in addition to the original four pilot cities, ten cities were already developing their own project or had expressed a strong commitment to do so. By mid-1992, Queensland and South Australia had statewide projects with state co-ordinators whose brief was to encourage existing and potential healthy cities and communities to develop their ideas. The funding for the pilot project ceased in mid-1990. A further two years' funding was provided to develop further the national network. The executive of this project comprised membership from three organizations: ACHA, the Local Government Association of Australia, and the Commission for the Future. This chapter reports on the research and evaluation activity that was conducted in Noarlunga during the period of the pilot project.

Noarlunga is an outer suburb of Adelaide, capital city of South Australia – the driest state in the driest continent. The state is known for its world-class wine, the biannual Festival of Arts, the Grand Prix, and its progressive liberal tradition that still exerts a strong influence on the state's direction and atmosphere. The state has been governed by Labor administrations for twenty years apart from a short period of Liberal government in the early 1980s.

Noarlunga is wedged between the urban sprawl to the north, some of the best vineyards in Australia to the east and spectacular coastal areas of long, sandy beaches interspersed by dramatic red cliffs to the west. The population of approximately 75,000 is projected to grow to over 130,000 by the year 2000. Noarlunga has experienced rapid population growth since its beginning as little more than a village in the early 1970s. Typical of many other communities on the outskirts of Australian cities, it is mortgage-belt territory with a high proportion of families with children – a third of the population is under fifteen. Noarlunga is characterized by tracts of detached housing on quarter-acre blocks. By European standards, the city sprawls: its main focus is the civic centre with its undercover shopping, council chambers, college of technical and further education, health services and offices of other government departments.

Noarlunga has provided a good political and social policy environment for the Healthy Cities project. Through the late 1980s, the South Australian Labour Government committed itself to a public policy approach to improving the health of South Australians. The primary health care policy, endorsed in 1990, has three aims: achieving equity in health status and in access to basic health care; promoting health and preventing illness; and reducing and controlling health service costs. This policy, together with the state's social justice strategy (which aims to reduce inequity by promoting a co-ordinated approach across government portfolios), has led to a climate supportive of projects which reflect new public health thinking. Regrettably, this climate became less rosy under the strains of the economic recession than it was during the life of the pilot project.

In addition to the supportive state environment, Noarlunga was fortunate in providing a sound basis for developing the Healthy Cities idea. A Community Services Forum had been established in 1980 and, through its monthly meetings, provided an opportunity for state government, council and community services and group representatives to exchange information, plan common strategies and lobby for additional resources for community initiatives. This group proved to be very supportive of the Healthy Cities project. Noarlunga also had three agencies funded by the State Health Commission: a women's health centre, a community health centre (both of which are managed by locally appointed boards of management) and a community-based research unit. These organizations had a strong commitment to health promotion and illness-prevention. A social planning team was established in 1984 to steer the social aspects of the newly developing suburbs in Noarlunga. This group comprised representatives from local government, welfare, health, transport, education, housing and the general community. Thus the notion of inter-sectoral collaboration had taken root in Noarlunga before the Healthy Cities project began.

After the project had been running for a year, its aims were modified to reflect developments in its operation. The modified aims were:

- to involve government agencies, non-government organizations and other sectors in the development of local health policies and actions which seek to establish a social, economic and physical environment conducive to health
- to implement the Healthy Cities project in a way that defines and promotes equity of access to the resources necessary to maintain good health and improve poor health
- to increase community awareness of social perspectives on health, in particular the social determinants of illness
- to encourage local health services' reorientation towards health promotion
- to implement and evaluate demonstration projects focusing on inter-sectoral co-operation and community involvement
- to evaluate the process and the outcome of the Healthy Cities project at the local level, using a common national framework

RESEARCH AND THE NEW PUBLIC HEALTH

In Australia, as in other countries, debate about appropriate science for public and community health research has continued since the 1970s. Some laboratory-based scientists have claimed epidemiologists are not proper scientists and some epidemiologists make the same claim about social scientists. The latter have taken a more prominent role in public health research in the past decade and argue that their methodologies and approaches to research have much to offer the understanding of public health. Experience has shown this to be the case, particularly in the areas of assessing needs and evaluation (Furler 1979; Owen and Mohr 1986; Feurstein 1986; Wadsworth 1988, 1991; Southern Community Health Research Unit (SCHRU) 1991).

At the heart of the methodological debate has been the question of whether a form of science designed for laboratory conditions can be adapted to study human society in its natural setting. The hallmark of good laboratory science is the ability to control sufficient factors to be able to arrive at definitive statements about cause and effect. It is very rarely that this is possible in natural settings. Societies and communities within them are complex. There are so many factors that might have an impact on the variables in the study that controlling for all of them generally becomes an impossibility. In any case, a social scientist would argue, it is not just the outcome of any experiment that is useful, but also the process of arriving there.

The complexities of the social world usually mean that a public health researcher will have to use other forms of science to come to grips with the topic of their study. Usually they will beat a path between a variety of methods and strive to ensure that these can cope with the less-than-tidy world of the average community. Wadsworth (1988) suggests that what is needed is engaged interaction with the social world. She maintains that researchers need to engage in experiential encounters which will enable them to grasp people's perceptions and understand what social phenomena mean to them. Reductionist thinking is rarely helpful and is not a strong approach when applied to community settings. The research related to Healthy Cities Noarlunga attempted to avoid this difficulty. If there was one guiding rule for the research it was that methods were selected to provide the information required, not because of any inherent commitment to a particular method.

THE CONTRIBUTION OF RESEARCH TO THE HEALTHY CITIES NOARLUNGA PILOT PROJECT

The research for Healthy Cities Noarlunga was undertaken by the Southern Community Health Research Unit (SCHRU). This unit was established in 1984 by the South Australian Health Commission. In 1992, the unit was amalgamated with its counterpart, the Northern Community Health Research Unit to form the South Australian Community Research Unit, with a widened mandate and a smaller budget. Its original brief was to research the health needs in the southern metropolitan area of Adelaide, to evaluate community health services and provide relevant social and demographic data to community health centres in its region. The unit is responsible to an advisory committee which consists of representatives from local health services. It has had independence from the central bureaucracy. Until 1990 the unit was based adjacent to a community health centre in Noarlunga. It was then well placed to conduct research relevant to the aims of a Healthy Cities project. Part of the research was undertaken before the Healthy Cities project came to Noarlunga. The rest was developed in conjunction with the Healthy Cities project. There were three categories of research activity:

1 Assessing needs: The Southern Community Health Research Unit chose Noarlunga as the first area in which to conduct a needs assessment for two reasons: the city's rapid population growth and the decision of the South Australian Health Commission to build a Health Village there. The needs assessment exercise aimed at providing data for planning the direction of this new Health Village.
2 Evaluation of the process of the pilot Healthy Cities project
3 The development of social indicators relating to the health status of the community, this included the collation of both qualitative and quantitative indicators.

The focus of the needs assessment done before the project was a community health survey conducted in mid-1985 with a sample randomly selected from the electoral roll. Questionnaires were posted to 2,066 residents, and 74 per cent (n = 1,495) responded. Two questionnaires were posted: one, respondents completed about themselves; the other sought information about any children the respondent might have and about his or her experience as a parent. The adult questionnaire was divided into five sections. The first covered health and illness and included the Nottingham Health Profile (Hunt *et al.* 1986b); the second collected socio-demographic data and information about the respondent's social networks; the third requested information on whether the respondent cared for anyone who was intellectually or physically disabled or psychiatrically ill; the fourth section dealt with recent life experiences such as bereavement and marriage; and the final section asked about the use of health and other community services. The questionnaire contained some open-ended questions which encouraged the respondents to express their opinions about the community.

The data from this survey have been widely used throughout the Noarlunga community. The survey's findings were reported to the community in a variety of ways as described below. Some general lessons can be drawn from this needs assessment work. Discussion of these will highlight the approach and the methods that were used.

A review of the literature on needs assessment conducted when the Noarlunga research began in 1985 indicated that while need had become a crucial factor in decision-making on resource allocation, the process of assessing need was fraught with conceptual and methodological challenges. It seemed as if needs studies were promoted as symbols of rationality, responsibility and democracy, while in practice they were not equipped to ensure these qualities (Ife 1980; Baum 1986). The Noarlunga exercise was designed to overcome some of the problems identified with earlier needs assessments. The principles developed in the Noarlunga exercise have subsequently been refined in further needs assessments (Baum and Abbott 1989; Kalucy 1989) and documented in a manual for use by community health workers (Southern Community Health Research Unit 1991). In summary, these principles are to define the difference between a problem and a solution; to clarify the values of the research team and those contributing to the research; and to have a community input. Each of these is considered in turn.

First, need is often equated with both a social or health problem and a prescription to solve that problem. This means that people may arrive at a solution to their problem without considering fully a range of solutions. Teachers and health workers may, for instance, conclude that parents in their community need parenting skill classes. This conclusion might be based on observation of what the professional workers define as undesirable parenting practice. An alternative view might be that there is a value difference between the professional workers and local parents' beliefs about parenting and that the professionals need training to understand reasons for local beliefs about parenting. Yet another view is that the parents need other supports for their parenting role such as improved public transport, more opportunities for social contact or, if they are living on a low income, more income.

In relation to health, professionals will often see needs in terms of their own skills (Illich 1977). Thus the solution for the widespread prevalence of backache in the community might be seen differently by chiropractors, physiotherapists, orthopaedic surgeons and yoga teachers.

The Noarlunga exercise indicated that one of the important roles a needs assessment should perform was encouraging lateral thinking about health problems among community members and health professionals. The data collected should be used to challenge existing beliefs. An example of this process in action was a workshop run as part of Health Issues Day that encouraged participants (community and health workers) to consider the question 'What makes you sick? You or your environment?' The workshop presented data from the Noarlunga Community Health Survey showing a relationship between living in a low-income household and reported health status. Participants were encouraged to reflect on possible explanations for this association.

Second, value judgements creep into all stages of needs assessment – from the decision of what area of need to investigate, to determining what actions should be taken to solve any given problem. In the Noarlunga study, the framework used by the research team was informed by an understanding of the social basis of health status. This framework was endorsed by a policy commitment to such an approach, enshrined in the South Australian Social Health Strategy document. The introduction to this states:

> A social view of health is one that recognizes the impact (both direct and indirect) that physical, socio-economic and cultural aspects of the environment have on the health of the community. A social view of health implies that we must intervene to change those aspects of the environment which are promoting ill health, rather than continue to simply deal with illness after it appears, or continue to exhort individuals to change their attitudes and lifestyles when, in fact, the environment in which they live and work gives them little choice or support for making such changes.
>
> (South Australian Health Commission, 1988)

This framework also includes a commitment to the pursuit of equity in health status. This commitment plays a role in determining that the distribution of health in a community across different groups should be an important focus of the needs assessment. The Noarlunga experience suggested that the adoption of such a framework was useful when analysing data and preparing reports. Users of the report may not necessarily agree with the framework but are given an understanding of the researchers' position. Values should not be ignored (they will not go away) and their clarification can assist planning and strategy development based on data from a needs assessment.

Third, limitations of relying on a professional health worker's views of the world have been noted. Obviously, specialists in any field have a considerable amount of expertise to offer to a needs assessment. The experts on the needs of a local community or a particular group within it should include those people who live and/or work in that community. Community involvement has long been advocated as desirable in a diverse range of government activities, including town planning and the management of health services. Experience suggests that achieving an effective community input is more difficult than the rhetoric often suggests (Sandercock 1978; Dixon 1989; Baum 1990). Bureaucracies and professional groups may manipulate the notion of community involvement so that the participation is in name only. Community members are generally in a less powerful position than those consulting them. As Dwyer (1989) noted: 'It is unrealistic to expect people to put energy into arrangements which are ineffective or have been invested with little or no power, or which are stacked against the community representatives.'

This realization may make people sceptical about participating in activities driven by government or other official agencies. Some researchers have tended to see community members as fodder for their research. Wadsworth (1984) has described the activities of much research as 'data raids' in which people provide information and then never hear of the researcher again. Understandably, this might lead to some cynicism about research and its benefits. In Noarlunga, attempts were made to increase the input of the community to the research process. The questionnaire used for the random community health survey included some questions that gave participants a chance to express their opinions. Many took advantage of this. The findings of the research were reported to the community in a report written in non-technical language and containing photographs and clear graphics. This publication has been in great demand throughout the Noarlunga community, especially by human service agencies and community groups. Following publication of the report, a Health Issues Day was held to report the main findings and encourage locals to participate in workshops to discuss the implications of the findings – moving the research from the problem-identification to the problem-solution stage. This day attracted 100 residents and fifty people who were employed in Noarlunga. The day encouraged the use of the research findings as a basis for local planning. The impact of the research was subtle and its ripples have been felt in planning for health and other community services and planning for the new areas of development in Noarlunga where green field sites are being developed into residential suburbs. An important impact of the research has been in providing information that supports an interpretation of health in a social context. Thus the data that highlighted differences in health status depending on gender, employment status, housing tenure and income have enriched the debate on health equity in Noarlunga.

It is a not uncommon observation that research findings are frequently left on the proverbial dusty shelf. This did not happen in Noarlunga. The reason why can be partly explained by the efforts made to listen to community input and facilitate occasions when the survey data were presented and discussed. The fact that the research was conducted by a research unit that was established on a permanent basis also helped ensure that the data found their way into planning decisions. Possibly the most important factor was that Noarlunga had a community services forum which brought together representatives from human services agencies, community groups and local state and federal politicians in the region. The forum which meets monthly and organizes many subcommittees was able to disseminate the research and contribute to its development. It also made a fertile seed bed for the Healthy Cities philosophy when it first arrived in Noarlunga.

Data from the community needs assessment formed an important part of the submission for funding for the Australian Healthy Cities Project. When the funding was granted, Noarlunga already had a body of data relating to its health status and the project's management committee was able to continue the process of identifying health problems and developing solutions to these. Healthy Cities was also able to work with the Southern Community Health Research Unit and continue the research process. This approach is more useful than a one-off survey and consultation. Continuity and development of the research helps increase the chances that it will be used.

The European Healthy Cities project agreed on a set of indicators that would provide a measure of the health status of a city. The Australian project followed suit. The initial intention was to agree on a set of indicators that could be collected for each city. In the event, each city approached the task a little differently. Noarlunga relied on the community health survey described above, mapped socio-economic data derived from census and other sources, data from the *South Australian Social Health Atlas* that permitted comparison to be made between Noarlunga and other local government areas in South Australia, and data collected as part of an Environmental Health Management Planning process. This latter exercise was co-ordinated by a committee with representatives from the local council, the Southern Community Health Research Unit, the Southern District Environment Group, Healthy Cities and the Public and Environmental Health section of the South Australian Health Commission. It built on the community health survey and covered topics that had not been included in that exercise. Some additional survey work was done to find out what community perceptions were by asking the question 'What do you believe are the three most important things that could make Noarlunga more healthy?' Responses to this question suggested that the randomly selected residents put most value on the physical and social environment, followed closely by the provision of a range of local services, as making a contribution to the city's health. Lifestyles were given much less emphasis. These results were interpreted as indicating community support for a social perspective on health (Cooke and Skewes 1990). The Environmental Health Plan also involved a consultation with key people in the community such as school principals and community service staff. The findings were pulled together in a draft report that was published by Healthy Cities in May 1990. This is being used as a basis for further environmental action by the Healthy Cities committee and the local council and health services. One example of this action is a council project to monitor the handling of chemicals in local industries.

The collection of mapped indicators (Table 8.1) has been used by a range of government agencies and community groups in Noarlunga. The maps are coloured and provide an effective means of showing the distribution of particular characteristics within the city. When the maps were first produced, workshops were run for managers and workers in government agencies and community-based organizations. These workshops presented the data and were then structured to encourage participants to reflect on their potential use and their limitations.

When the indicator data were presented to the Healthy Cities management committee there was some disquiet expressed by the community members at the notion of stigmatizing areas that continually rated highly on indicators of disadvantage such as high unemployment, larger than average proportion of government housing, single parents and people on low incomes. For professional workers, in contrast, these indicators were viewed as a means of implementing a social justice element to planning services and other initiatives. The community members believed that focusing on the negative aspects of any particular area ran the risk of giving the area a bad name and making life worse for the residents. In response to this the Southern Community Health Research Unit decided to conduct a detailed study of one of the areas that rated highly on indicators of disadvantage. The report that resulted relied on observation, detailed

Table 8.1   Noarlunga: some quantitative social indicators

Demography
    Fertility, births and deaths
    Age breakdown of the population
Social indicators of well-being
    Marital status
    Single parents
    Proficiency with the English language
    Low incomes
    Housing
    Private cars
    Unemployed people
    Women's labour force participation
    Occupational groups
Illness indicators
    Hospital separations
    Mortality
    Sexually transmitted disease

Note: This information was presented in a series of maps produced using computer graphics.
Source: Southern Community Health Research Unit (1989)

interviewing of health and social service workers, residents and local leaders such as the minister and councillors, and showed that, while the area did have more than its share of disadvantage, there were also some considerable strengths. The qualitative methodology enabled a range of perceptions, feelings and stories about the suburb to emerge that described, more fully than the statistical data, the health and well-being experienced. The following section from the report illustrates this:

> One particularly powerful theme to emerge during the research was the strength of character of some local people. Some service providers described how some less advantaged individuals and groups have responded to situations of pressure by developing particular resources ... Positive characteristics named by some service providers included liveliness, honesty, perseverance, spontaneity, optimism, a commitment to their children, energy, persistence at working to make ends meet and pride in achievements.
>
> (Traynor 1990: 47)

This report put into practice Hancock and Duhl's (1986) advice that, 'Unless data are turned into stories that can be understood by all, they are not effective in any process of change, either political or administrative.'

EVALUATION OF THE PILOT PROJECT

Evaluation was considered an important part of the Healthy Cities Australia Pilot Project because the funding body had made it a condition of funding, and because those who submitted the original application for the funding were committed to evaluation as a means of understanding and improving programmes. The approach to evaluation advocated at the outset of the project has been documented (Baum and Brown 1989) and was more or less followed throughout the pilot project. This approach was based on a commitment to conducting evaluation that was useful to the key stakeholders in the project and which selected the most appropriate methodology to provide this information. The Healthy Cities Australia National Executive established a research and evaluation subgroup which co-ordinated the evaluation between the three pilot cities and worked with the external evaluator who was contracted at the end of the project to synthesize the city evaluations and provide a commentary on the progress of the national project (Worsley 1990).

Often, when the question of methodology has been raised in relation to the evaluation, commentators, particularly those from a biomedical perspective, have advocated the use of a control city method to assess the impact of Healthy Cities on the population's health. This suggestion was considered inappropriate for two reasons. First, the Healthy Cities pilot project was modestly funded for only three years and could not reasonably be expected to have immediate measurable impacts on health status. Second, it was considered unlikely that Noarlunga could be matched in any meaningful way. While there are local government areas in South Australia similar to Noarlunga in some respects, there are many more ways in which they are different. There would be no way of knowing whether any observed differences were a result of the Healthy Cities project or the difference between the communities. In any case, interest in the Healthy Cities project was more to do with the processes of social change, and the quasi-experimental design did not offer much hope of furthering understanding in this area. This view was supported by the growing literature critical of the application of methods that are powerful in a laboratory setting, but which lose much of their meaningfulness when applied to a community (Furler 1989; Owen and Mohr 1986; Nutbeam and Catford 1987; Feurstein 1986).

The approach adopted in Noarlunga then, strove to provide a holistic understanding of the project's progress and achievements, and to monitor its subtle aspects. It was as important to know why the project succeeded or failed as to whether it did. It was recognized that communities are dynamic, unpredictable and extremely complex. The evaluation methods chosen were those that promised to do some justice to the variety of perspectives, understandings and events that contributed to the pilot project (Baum *et al.* 1990). The complexities of the social world ensured that the data would be messy and sometimes conflicting. But the evaluation method gave the best chance of making sense of a project that relied on interaction, conflict and development among people and organizations. An additional advantage was that as the evaluation focused on the project's process, its findings were able to be used to refine the project as it progressed.

The evaluation started with the assumption that values were an integral part of the development of the project and the interpretations of its progress. Those connected with a project such as Healthy Cities are unlikely to share common beliefs of interpretation of events. It was accepted that the picture of Healthy Cities which would be portrayed would need to incorporate varying views and that, at times, these would conflict with each other. The evaluator who ignores these values and political differences does so at the risk of missing out dimensions of the project which are its lifeblood.

The Noarlunga evaluation collected information on the following topics:

- policy changes
- collaboration between different sectors in services provision and planning
- planning
- community involvement and awareness
- changes in the way local public service workers approached their work
- perceptions of key stakeholders' perceptions of the project.

The methods were chosen to fit the available resources and the evaluation approach discussed in the previous section. They were:

- key informant interviews (face-to-face during the early stages of the project and again in the concluding stages)
- audit of attendance at meetings of committee members
- questionnaire surveys of key groups:
  - management and reference committee members
  - local health and education workers
  - local community (to assess the project)
- analysis of local media
- documentation of additional resources attracted to the project

– ongoing monitoring of the project by members of the research team who played an active role in Noarlunga Healthy Cities

These various sources of information were used to build up a picture of the pilot project.

The results of the evaluation of the Noarlunga project have been reported more fully elsewhere (Baum *et al.* 1990; Baum and Cooke 1992). Here, selected findings will be used to demonstrate the ways in which the evaluation was able to elucidate certain issues and contribute to the project's development.

An important aspect of the evaluation was monitoring the development of particular projects in which community action was supported by professional workers. An issue that emerged from the data collected in the early stages of the project was criticism that Healthy Cities was colonizing existing initiatives. In response to this, the evaluators, in consultation with the project management committee, identified three types of project: those for which Healthy Cities took an initiating role and which remained Healthy Cities initiatives; those for which Healthy Cities took a key role initially but withdrew; and projects where Healthy Cities supported an existing community group, exercise, issue or initiative.

One of the exciting projects initiated by Healthy Cities was the Visions of Noarlunga.

Noarlunga 2000 and Beyond. Visions of a healthy Noarlunga – you are invited to share your ideas and visions for the future of Noarlunga

So ran the advertisement in the local *Messenger Press* for this Community Forum and Fun Day in October 1989. This project, which was first conceived as a community booklet, blossomed into a community arts event with funding from the South Australian Department for the Arts, Noarlunga Council and Noarlunga Health Service with its own artist in residence and project photographer. The day was the culmination of a year's research in the form of community Visions of a Healthy City workshops. This climax, which included the production by community groups of nearly one hundred images of a healthy Noarlunga, resulted in the construction of the Dream Machine – a wooden framework holding a number of moving two-and-three dimensional images. The Dream Machine has subsequently been on tour to schools and community centres.

Five key informants provided information about this project and all felt that it was either successful or very successful. All considered that Healthy Cities contributed a great deal to it and thought it either unlikely or very unlikely that the project would have been developed without Healthy Cities involvement.

Two key informants cited Visions as an example of successful community and inter-agency involvement. It was

> a focus that the community could identify with, to take their issues and talk them through ... strengthening of a clearer identity for Noarlunga.

One informant saw Visions as an energy-raising project:

> Idealism and vision is energizing some health workers, especially Visions workshop. Stimulates more optimistic thought.

Most key informants identified community involvement and consciousness-raising as the first steps in bringing about change. Visions enabled

> the community to look forward and to identify what they would like to see in the future and therefore what changes would need to be made. For community to identify with the area – to have a feeling of ownership of their environment.

The desired results included 'some fun' – an underrated energizing force – and the starting of a process in Noarlunga to

> contribute to the cultural life of the area with something that can be built upon... I hoped to be part of a chain reaction and give people a taste of what it is like to be involved in the arts.

Healthy Cities was seen by all as initiator and facilitator, providing background research and administrative and emotional support. It was also seen as successfully attracting necessary funding. Extra funding would have enabled Healthy Cities to make this a more effective project by widening its scope in terms of time, and as an ongoing project.

The following factors were seen by informants to facilitate the project:

- an existing close-knit community in Noarlunga at large and among those involved in the project
- widespread enthusiasm for the project
- it was innovative which helped it gain funding
- there was community and agency support
- Healthy Cities was a skilled and successful co-ordinator of the project

Most respondents felt that the lack of resources – particularly financial – was the only factor that hindered the project. One person involved felt that the two-month interregnum between Healthy Cities project managers in 1989 caused some confusion and tension within the project.

One respondent felt that the community arts movement was not only a powerful method of raising issues, but an appropriate one for Healthy Cities:

> It can help people understand what Healthy Cities was all about. The art form conveyed possibly threatening concepts in a non-threatening way. I would like to see Healthy Cities carry on a connection with community arts. It has been good for the community arts movement. Healthy Cities and the community arts movement make good allies.

Another project in the pilot period rated as successful by the evaluation process was the campaign to clean up the Onkaparinga Estuary. The quality of the water in the Onkaparinga Estuary had been an issue in Noarlunga for twenty years and surveys of this water undertaken during this time had found high bacterial levels. Estuary water has been polluted by two main sources – agricultural and industrial activities and urban development. Fertilizers from farming and effluent from Metro Meat Abattoirs drained into the river as did storm water run-off from the expanding southern housing areas in Noarlunga. The pollution, coupled with limited natural flushing from the tides, resulted in bacterial levels that, according to studies done by the South Australian Department of Environment and Planning and the Engineering & Water Supply Department, were higher than would be regarded as safe to swim in. All of this was frequently reported in the local newspaper.

Several groups were formed to tackle the pollution problems. The Noarlunga Council set up a working party in 1988 and Noarlunga Healthy Cities became involved via the Environmental Health Management Plan. Public meetings were called by Healthy Cities from March 1989 to discuss the pollution problems and possible solutions. The need for intersectoral action was highlighted at the first of these meetings where it emerged that five government agencies had jurisdiction over different aspects of the river. This had resulted in the situation where none of the agencies would accept responsibility for dealing with the pollution. Two developments came from the public meetings: the Onkaparinga Estuary Water Quality Group, with wide representation, was formed; and the Minister of Water Resources and Lands announced in May 1989 that a task force, comprising state and local government representatives, would be formed to address the problem. A report with recommendations was released in 1990.

Five key informants answered questions on the Onkaparinga Estuary campaign and had close involvement with one of the groups tackling the pollution problem. They became involved in the project for various reasons, three of them because they valued the river and wanted it cleaned up and preserved, another in a professional capacity as health surveyor, and the fifth as a representative of Healthy Cities.

One informant felt that the key issue was

> getting the Government to get its finger out – getting all parties together including other Councils to develop sensible Supplementary Development Plans and farming practices.

All informants hoped that their involvement would result in action – that the community would be made more aware of the problems and that the river would be cleaned up – and all believed that their hopes had either been realized or that significant progress had been made. All of the informants, except one, rated the project as either successful or very successful. The others rated it as neither successful nor unsuccessful. All informants thought that Healthy Cities had contributed a lot to the project. Healthy Cities' role was seen primarily as providing a resource and co-ordination function as well as one of advocacy on behalf of the community groups. Healthy Cities

> opened all the doors that needed opening. Ministers, etc. took notice of Healthy Cities, wouldn't have taken notice of individuals or the community.

One informant saw the Healthy Cities role differently to the others. It contributed a

> potential watch-dog/surveillance in the interests of the public.

All but one of the informants considered that Healthy Cities could not have been any more effective than it was, though one believed that Healthy Cities could have taken a higher profile. Informants considered that Healthy Cities' involvement and political support were the two major factors that helped address the issue. One informant believed that the increasing awareness of environmental issues was an important contributing factor.

Hindering factors mentioned by the informants related to the role of government (both state and local) – too many departments involved but none of them taking responsibility, inflexibility of the Engineering and Water Supply Department, and lack of local government commitment. Only two informants mentioned other supports that may have helped – the government following up on earlier reports on the state of the river, and support from councils upstream. Two informants expressed the hope that a body would be formed to take responsibility for the issue in the future (one specifically mentioned Healthy Cities as this body).

These two case-studies of Healthy Cities projects provide an indication of the monitoring that was done as part of the evaluation. Findings from case-studies of this type were reviewed and a series of factors that helped or hindered community projects was derived. These were discussed and refined with the Healthy Cities management committee. The factors are summarized in Table 8.2.

The evaluation, as well as looking at particular projects, also aimed to investigate the process underlying Healthy Cities initiatives. The data from the evaluation suggest that the relationship between the Healthy Cities project and local community health workers was not always smooth. The project aimed to reorient local health services towards health promotion. The local health service was, until 1990 when a hospital was built, a large community health service employing 100 people. A study, conducted in 1985, of the activities and attitudes of community health workers in Noarlunga had identified a significant gap between the policy statements of the local services (which strongly endorsed health promotion) and actual practice (Southern Community Health Services Research Unit (SCHSRU) 1987). A follow-up study done in 1987 (SCHSRU 1988) showed that the reported work practices of community health workers had become more directed to prevention. Thus before the Healthy Cities project started there was evidence that the reorientation was already happening.

Health workers were surveyed at the start and finish of the project. These surveys showed that there was quite strongly divided opinion amongst the health workers in terms of their evaluation of the benefits of the Healthy Cities project. The evaluators concluded after the first survey that Healthy Cities had won few converts but was encouraging those who were already working in a community development mode. One of the resentments that emerged at the beginning of the project was that some health workers believed that Healthy Cities was claiming credit for their achievements. In response to this, the Healthy Cities project team took care to acknowledge who had been responsible for initiatives they quoted as models of good practice. At the time of the second survey, this polarization was still present. Most of the health workers who responded to the survey claimed not to have a great deal of knowledge of the project and that it had not had much effect on their work or the work of their team or centre. For some, this was because they felt they already operated in the way Healthy Cities advocated. For others, it signalled a critical attitude to the project. Some saw Healthy Cities as elitist or empire building and expressed resentment at the resources allocated to it.

Health workers who were more positive to Healthy Cities (about

Table 8.2 Helping and hindering forces in the Healthy Cities projects

Helping	Hindering
Close community – commitment from a cadre of community members. Community awareness increasing and people willing to attend public meetings	Community involvement limited in some instances. The social action approach (bottom–up) may conflict with a social planning approach (top–down)
Clearly defined objectives and desired outcome	Not always possible from an original good idea that needs to 'mature'
Healthy Cities assists with resources	Inadequate resources – help in kind to community groups but no financial support
Healthy Cities provides legitimacy to some community action and encourages other agencies to participate	The perceived radicalism of some community groups may make established agencies and local and state government departments wary of the Healthy Cities idea. This may reduce Healthy Cities credibility with some agencies
Healthy Cities was an excellent vehicle for community expression of needs	
Healthy Cities was perceived to be neutral and so was able to facilitate participation from a number of sectors	Concern over the future of the Healthy Cities project reduced its credibility
Healthy Cities was able to engender enthusiasm	Healthy Cities had no formal power (other than of ideas) or resources with which to influence agencies
Many Healthy Cities initiatives reflected and complemented the growing tide of green awareness	Bureaucratic responses can dampen enthusiasm and some issues
	Many of these issues are hard to resolve and should be expected to take a long time to resolve

Source: Baum *et al*. (1990)

one-third of those responding to the survey) identified a number of positive benefits they believed the project had: it encouraged creative approaches to health promotion, legitimized a social approach to health, encouraged more co-operation across sectors and provided useful resources. A typical positive comment was:

> the Healthy Cities approach is part of, and sets the scene for, the broader community health concepts. Healthy Cities has helped to establish the philosophy and do some of the ground work in this area.

Another theme that came out of the evaluation data in regard to the local health services involvement with Healthy Cities was that of how close the involvement should be. The project was located in the Noarlunga Health Village and a number of respondents in the final evaluation felt that it may, as a consequence, have become too closely identified with the health sector, particularly at the expense of its links with local government. The final report concluded that the project would benefit from a location that was not identified solely with any one government agency.

These examples show the value of evaluation data to developing and analysing the complexities of Healthy Cities. Further details are available in the final report (Baum *et al.* 1990).

CONCLUSION

The Noarlunga Healthy Cities project was fortunate in having available the support of a community health research unit. The unit had conducted relevant needs assessment research before the project began, continued this work during the project and was well-equipped to develop appropriate methodologies for the evaluation. The systematic approach to research and evaluation had a number of benefits for the Healthy Cities project. The impact of the research was subtle and contributed to fine-tuning the project in various ways.

The development of the project in Noarlunga was a case of muddling through, guided by the overall objectives. This was inevitable if Healthy Cities was to be responsive to its stakeholders' ideas and to changing circumstances (for example capitalizing on the rapid growth in community interest in environmental concerns). The evaluation strategy was flexible enough to adapt to this muddling through because it had been designed with that eventuality in mind. The final report, as a result, was able to tell a story that took this messiness into account not as an annoying contaminating variable, but as part of the essential life-blood of the project.

The evaluation encouraged critical appraisal of the developing Healthy Cities projects. There is a danger, common to many new and visionary projects, that those involved in them become so immersed that they lose their perspective of their endeavour. This is particularly the case when the project has to be marketed as a good idea. Regular reports from the evaluation team to the management committee guarded against this tendency. They also allowed time for assessment and reflection on the project's process. This was particularly true of the time spent on evaluation at each of the eight national workshops. Each pilot city would have a chance to report on activities and this would result in informal assessment.

In Noarlunga, the insider nature of the evaluation encouraged this reflection. Appraisal of health promotion projects like Healthy Cities is important in terms of acceptability to those groups with an investment in it, particularly those who had invested resources.

The research activity proved to be educative. Conducting the needs assessment exercise encouraged those involved to challenge their existing ideas and provided resources that could be used in planning over a number of years. Researchers were challenged about their reliance on hard social indicators by members of particular communities who could offer an experiential perspective that was also of value to understanding communities. The learning that happens in the course of research projects is often overlooked when the benefits of research are appraised. Sometimes research results are dismissed as obvious. Often that is because they have new insights that are indeed obvious but not until they are actually pointed out. A well-conducted evaluation usually should not, by the end of the process, come as any great surprise to the various stakeholders. If it has been conducted in a collaborative way that takes account of the different values and perspectives of those involved in the initiative being evaluated, and provides for input from representatives of the main stakeholders, then it is likely to produce useful results.

The evaluation has had a number of audiences. Some of these have been interested in it in terms of acceptability for the resources invested in it. It seems particularly important that initiatives like Healthy Cities, based on relatively untried approaches involving community people and co-operation across sectors, should be closely monitored so that a knowledge base is developed for others exploring similar territory. People from other communities within Australia and beyond have been able to use the evaluation report to develop their own projects and ideas. The evaluation has contributed to theoretical knowledge about health promotion. An example of this was in developing understanding about the nature, extent and effectiveness of community involvement. The evaluation data brought out the gap between policy statements about community participation and the actuality of bringing it about. The picture of community participation painted was more complex, showing that building effective partnerships between the community and paid professionals is no easy task. The report identified some of the challenges (such as ensuring that participation is not just a token gesture that doesn't really dilute professional modes of operation). Understanding the contradictions and challenges in the new public health is an important task for researchers. These insights make the research useful as a systematic documentation of what this, sometimes vague, concept of the new public health is about in practice.

ACKNOWLEDGEMENTS

Thanks are extended to Helma McHugh for her usual efficient and speedy word processing and to Norma McCarthy for her thorough proof-reading.

Chapter 9

Healthy Cities within the American context

Beverly C. Flynn

INTRODUCTION: THE CONTEXT

As successful as Healthy Cities has been in Europe and Canada, Healthy Cities in the United States is only one among several health promotion models that have emerged to support communities in their quest for improved community health. In the United States, states and local communities continue to have expanding responsibilities for meeting health needs without concomitant resources. At the same time, there are serious problems in public health, not the least the difficulties in adequately assuring the conditions in which people can be healthy (Institute of Medicine 1988). Many public health issues have become politicized and public health professionals lack the power needed to pursue essential programmes. Over the years there has not been a constituency for public health in the USA. On the positive side, there is national and local concern and a commitment to improving the public's health. Evidence of this may be seen in the development of community health promotion approaches which are discussed in this chapter.

There are people in America who are willing and accustomed to taking local action to solve problems. The concept of democracy aimed at self-sufficiency appeals to Americans. However, community leaders frequently do not understand or exercise their potential in community health promotion. Consistent with the pluralistic form of democracy present in the United States, a number of recently published benchmarks and approaches to community health promotion now exist to help communities involve the public in public health. These include Assessment Protocol for Excellence in Public Health (APEX/PH), Healthy Cities, Healthy Communities, Healthy Communities 2000, Model Standards, Planned Approach to Community Health (PATCH) and the National Health Promotion and Disease Prevention Objectives for the year 2000 (APEX/PH 1991; Flynn 1992; California Healthy Cities Project 1990;

National Civic League 1991; PATCH 1989; *Healthy People 2000, National Health Promotion and Disease Prevention Objectives* 1990).

THE NATIONAL OBJECTIVES

The national objectives cover 297 different aims for improving the health of Americans in the next ten years, and are organized in the following twenty-two priority areas:

- physical activity and fitness
- nutrition
- tobacco
- alcohol and other drugs
- family planning
- mental health and mental disorders
- violent and abusive behaviour
- educational and community-based programmes
- unintentional injuries
- occupational safety and health
- environmental health
- food and drug safety
- oral health
- maternal and infant health
- heart disease and stroke
- cancer
- diabetes and chronic disabling conditions
- HIV infection
- sexually transmitted diseases
- immunization and infectious diseases
- clinical preventive services
- surveillance and data systems

Although considerably more extensive, the national health objectives are comparable to the World Health Organization's (WHO) thirty-eight European targets. There are three overall goals for the national health objectives:

1 increase the span of healthy life for Americans
2 reduce health disparities among Americans
3 achieve access to preventive services for all Americans

As a spin-off from the Consensus Conference held in 1990 to discuss effects to improve public health, a guide was developed to describe the contribution of the variety of models to improving health at the local level, as measured by the national health objectives (Centers for Disease Control 1991). Figure 9.1 was prepared by the Centers for Disease Control as an overview of their conclusions following the conference. The areas of assessment, policy development and assurance were functions of local health departments recommended by the Institute of Medicine in their study of public health. The Centers for Disease Control concluded that the publication *Healthy Communities 2000: Model Standards* (1991), which is directly linked to the national health objectives, should be used by local health departments and the communities they serve as they formulate health outcome and process objectives. It also was concluded that APEX/PH was the only approach that assesses the agency's capacity to address public health in the community.

CURRENT MODELS OF COMMUNITY HEALTH PROMOTION IN THE UNITED STATES

Assessment Protocol for Excellence in Public Health (APEX/PH)

APEX/PH is a three-part, self-assessment process, guided by a manual, for use by local health departments to assess and improve their organizational capacity, to assess the health status of the community and actively to involve the community in improving community health. Part I of APEX/PH directs the user to develop and implement an action plan to improve the health department's organizational capacity in meeting the public health needs of the community, which could help to correct a deficit found by the Institute of Medicine's (1988) study on public health. Part II involves key members of the community in the assessment of community health needs and the identification of the role of the local health department in relation to community strengths and health problems. This results in the development of a community health plan for implementation which is data based, contains the input of the community and is accepted by the local health policy board. It is then that the national health objectives are considered for local relevance, and included in the plan. Part III discusses the policy development and assurance functions of the local health department, which also supports the recommendations of the Institute of Medicine's study on public health.

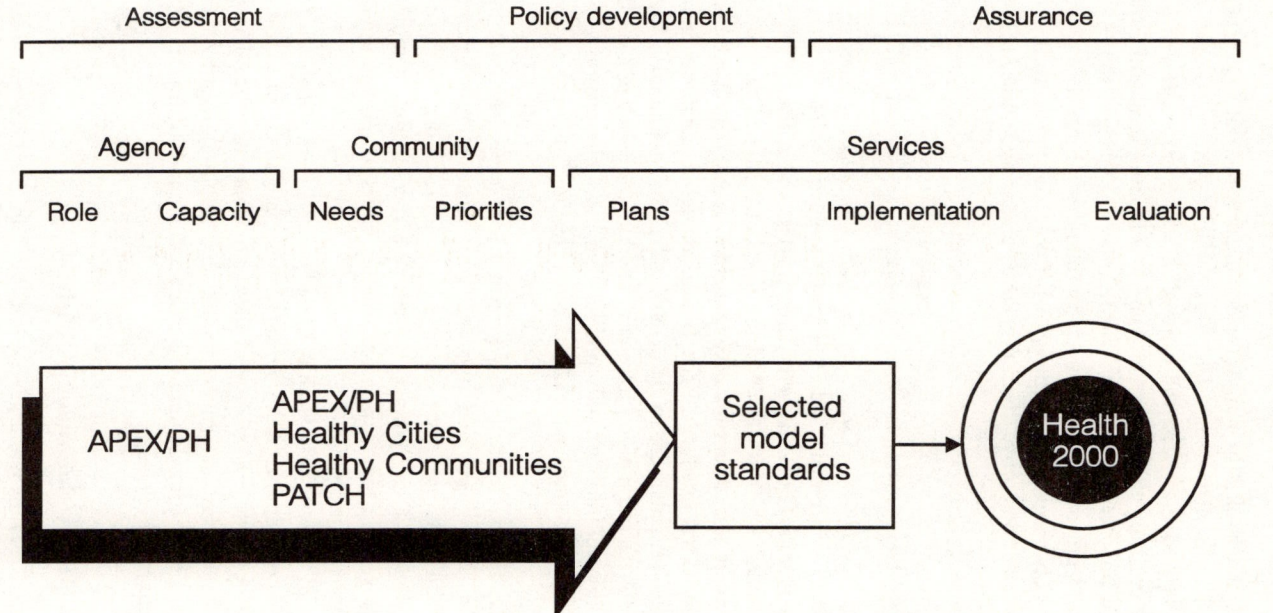

Figure 9.1 Targeting the year 2000
Source: United States Department of Health and Human Services, Public Health Service, Centers for Disease Control (December 1990)

Healthy Communities 2000: Model Standards

The latest guidebook is the companion document to the year 2000 national health objectives. It is designed to help public health professionals and community leaders translate the national objectives into state and local actions by focusing attention on assessing health status, setting objectives and formulating action strategies. The document also helps public health officials and other key members of communities negotiate and work co-operatively to ensure a partnership between the public and private sectors in order to improve the health, environment, and quality of life in communities.

Healthy Cities

Two statewide Healthy Cities projects have the longest history in the United States – in Indiana and California – and cities in other states are becoming Healthy Cities, including Boston, Mass. and Buffalo, N. Y. The Indiana model, which is described in more detail later in this chapter, involves community leadership development in community-based health promotion. Cities involved in the Indiana model conduct community assessments and a public debate about the health of the community, identify health problems and develop solutions, advocate for public policies that support the community's health, provide data-based information to pol-icy-makers and monitor and evaluate their Healthy Cities projects over time.

The California Healthy Cities project selects cities based on their submission of proposals and one-year work plans for implementing Healthy Cities pilot projects. Each city's commitment is demonstrated by the adoption of a city council resolution and a steering committee representative of the public and private sectors. Cities are selected annually to participate in the project.

Although the statewide Healthy Cities projects were initiated before the most recent national health objectives were published, the objectives have been found to cover many of the major concerns of the Healthy Cities. The national objectives can be used by local Healthy Cities Committees or steering groups in planning and monitoring local progress in addressing their concerns.

National Healthy Communities Initiative

The National Healthy Communities Initiative aimed to help communities design a collaborative, problem-solving process for creating a healthy community. The Healthy Communities Initiative indicated a link to the national health objectives and planned several approaches to stimulate healthy communities projects. A guide was developed which identified information resources that are available to healthy communities projects. The Healthy Communities Action Project assisted participants to implement Healthy Communities projects. The National Civic League has co-operated with the US Office of Disease Prevention and Health Promotion of the Public Health Service in accomplishing these objectives.

Planned Approach to Community Health (PATCH)

The PATCH programme is designed to help communities plan, implement and evaluate health promotion and health education programmes by working with representatives from the community, state and local health departments, and the Centers for Disease Control. PATCH mobilizes the community to participate in a community diagnosis and to identify community interventions and evaluation strategies. Although PATCH was developed before the year 2000 national health objectives, local community objectives can be found to parallel the national objectives. Mortality data, behavioural risk data and opinion information are collected every three years to monitor the health status of the community.

Clearly, all these models are indicative of local and/or national concern about the need to change the way community health is practised. All approaches involve community leaders in the decision-making process for improving the public's health. APEX/PH is the only model that focuses on assessing and improving the local health department's organizational capacity. *Healthy Communities 2000: Model Standards*, Healthy Cities Indiana, PATCH and APEX/PH include community participation in community assessments and establishing a community-wide health plan that is data based and facilitates implementation and evaluation. Healthy Cities Indiana and the California Healthy Cities project require local commitment and local Healthy Cities or steering committees to participate.

HEALTHY CITIES: THE INDIANA MODEL

Healthy Cities Indiana began in 1988 with a grant from the W. K. Kellogg Foundation as a collaborative effort between Indiana University School of Nursing, Indiana Public Health Association and six Indiana cities: Fort Wayne, Gary, Indianapolis, Jeffersonville, New Castle and Seymour. The

W. K. Kellogg Foundation supported the Healthy Cities Indiana project under their priority for community leadership development in community-oriented primary health care. In 1990, Healthy Cities Indiana became an integral part of the new Institute of Action Research for Community Health at Indiana University School of Nursing. As an action research project of the institute, Healthy Cities Indiana incorporates the following principles:

1 it is a joint effort of the researcher and community people – a co-operative activity
2 it involves systematic collection and analysis of information for the purposes of political action and social change

Consistent with Winter's (1987) definition of action research, Healthy Cities Indiana involves the integration of research, community participation and political action in public health. A brief description of Healthy Cities Indiana will facilitate the discussion of action research results to date.

Healthy Cities Indiana evolved out of experiences preparing graduate-level public health nurses in primary health care and health promotion to achieve the goal of Health for All by the year 2000. It was realized that preparing health professionals for public health practice was not enough. Problems facing local communities are much too complex to be resolved by health professionals alone. Community leaders also need to develop their skills in order to enter into local decision making about community health. Healthy Cities Indiana is an adaptation of the World Health Organization's Healthy Cities project in Europe and the Canadian Healthy Communities Project. In the United States, political authority is highly fractionalized and decentralized. While the government funds some health services, for the most part it only subsidizes the private health care delivery system, a private system that spends most of the health care resources on high technology sick care and, by comparison, very little on health promotion and disease prevention. Also, as noted earlier, public health in the United States has severe system difficulties. In Canada and in most of the countries in Europe there are more universal health care systems, more centralized political decision-making, and well organized public health systems.

Consistent with action research, in Healthy Cities Indiana, emphasis is placed on a community development approach to decision-making. Appropriate to the American context, Healthy Cities Indiana utilizes a community leadership development approach which helps local people critically re-examine the community in which they live and to increase their skill and involvement in solving community health problems. Community development is aimed at promoting local self-reliance (Schwartz 1982). Healthy Cities Indiana therefore:

- emphasizes placing health on the political agenda of the city
- requires community leaders to consider the health effects of their decisions
- views health broadly and as a shared responsibility of the entire community, not just the health professions
- focuses on hard-to-reach populations, the poor, minorities, children, elderly
- promotes healthy public policies.

These are integral to community leadership development.

This approach makes several assumptions about the milieu within which policy decisions are made in the United States. First, it assumes that the political system of elected representation operates imperfectly. A second assumption is that pluralism, while a means of increasing citizen participation, suffers from class and gender bias (Benz 1975). An additional assumption is that public policies are improved through broad-based participation in the policy-making process.

Healthy Cities Indiana uses a community development approach which builds on the strengths of the United States and the Midwest: self-reliance, the work ethic and a strong affinity for self-government. Healthy Cities Indiana seeks to assist local communities to develop leadership for broad-based solutions to today's complex health concerns. In addition to the development of leadership for health within the city, the Indiana model of Healthy Cities requires the following:

- city commitment demonstrated by both the local health officer and mayor
- establishment of a Healthy Cities committee that is broadly representative of the community as a whole
- community assessment and a public debate about the health of the community
- identification of health problems and development of solutions
- advocacy for public policies that support the community's health
- provision of data-based information to policy-makers, information which will support the development of healthy public policies
- monitoring and evaluating Healthy Cities projects over time

The Healthy Cities Committee in each city is the primary focus of the leadership development activities, although these activities are open to all interested community leaders. The committees were formed in 1988. The methods of community leadership development include: on-site consultation with Healthy Cities experts, technical support by project staff, local and statewide workshops which include training in vision workshops, analysing data and the meaning of data, establishing priorities and action plans, working with policy-makers and the media, proposal writing, national and international conferences, and networking across cities for shared learning. To facilitate the dissemination of information, the Healthy Cities Resource Center was established. The following are some of the resources that have been provided to each of the six Healthy Cities committees and are available, at cost, to others requesting them:

- introductory information on Healthy Cities
- video tapes
- audio tape
- bibliography on Healthy Cities
- books relevant to Healthy Cities
- consultation
- WHO Healthy Cities papers published by FADL, Copenhagen, Denmark

As noted earlier, Healthy Cities Indiana is an example of action research, a form of applied research. The purposes of action research in Healthy Cities is to promote informed action, enhance decision-making and apply knowledge to solve community health problems. Action research in Healthy Cities addresses five areas of impact:

- leadership development for community health
- dissemination of developed leadership
- development of action programmes for community health
- involvement of policy-makers in public health
- policy change

Both qualitative and quantitative methods of research are used, including minutes of Healthy Cities committee meetings, existing data, surveys, evaluation of workshops and network sessions by programme participants, the results of the Healthy Cities Committee Effectiveness Inventory which was completed by committee members, media reports and on-site observation by project directors and staff. These methods provide a wealth of information to the cities. Each of the five areas of impact will be discussed below, highlighting examples from the Healthy Cities.

How have the workshops, network sessions, consultations and technical support functioned to develop community leaders for public health? The statewide workshops and network sessions were well attended by four of the cities, who ranked them highly. The remaining two cities had representatives of the Healthy Cities committees attend the workshops. One of the cities participated strongly in workshops when they were on-site, but travel to statewide workshops was found to be difficult for committee members.

The results of the Healthy Cities Committee Effectiveness Inventory provided information to the committees that facilitated the leadership change (committee chair) in four cities, expanding committee membership in another city, developing more formal committee structures in three cities and establishing subcommittees or steering groups in all cities.

Consultation with staff led to the development of committee goals, objectives and priorities in all cities, and increased committee participation and functioning in several cities. In one large city, the vision workshop stimulated two neighbourhoods to participate in the Healthy Cities process. The result has been a parallel Healthy Cities process at the neighbourhood level, with representation of the neighbourhoods on the city-wide committee.

How have the Healthy Cities committee members used their leadership skills to further the health of their communities? Several examples provide evidence of leadership dissemination to the broader community. In one city, the first committee chair has become the local public health officer and he has retained the community-based view of public health. The educational representative on the Healthy Cities committee has become an advocate for youth health issues and co-ordinates the in-school, teen–parent programme sponsored by the committee. In this same city, the current chair has organized theologians to involve the churches in health. Realizing the potential impact on the county, the Healthy Cities committee has recently expanded its membership to include all cities and towns of the county.

In another city, two committee members serve on the state-mandated solid waste management district advisory committee. The chair of the committee was directly involved in developing a national survey of youth health needs. Two other committee members have taken an active role in the local redevelopment commission.

In another city the mayor, who was an active committee member, was elected to the state legislature. He co-authored bills on local scholarships, remedies for racial/sexual harassment, state-funded purchase of green spaces and land set-asides, and an expanded homemaker service programme for the elderly. Committee members have formed coalitions for child-abuse, indigent/homeless services and literacy. The committee as a whole assisted neighbouring towns to begin community walking programmes. Another example involves a member of the Healthy Cities committee who is a home economics teacher in a local high school. She was able to establish a community coalition to fund and operate a summer teen-parent programme in the school. The mayor of another city has not only been actively involved in supporting his city as a Healthy City but has participated in promoting Healthy Cities in the state and internationally. He has attended two WHO Healthy Cities Symposia in Europe and served as the vice chair of the congress in 1990.

What short-term projects and long-range programmes have been developed as a result of participation in Healthy Cities Indiana? Each of the cities has been involved in both short-term and long-range action strategies which have empowered the committees to take further action. Table 9.1 summarizes these strategies. In just a few years, the cities have been able, not only to initiate the Healthy Cities process, but also to develop multiple Healthy Cities projects that aim to improve the community's health.

How and to what extent, have local policy-makers been involved in the Healthy Cities process? The mayors or their staff and the local health department staff have actively participated in the Healthy Cities committee in all cities. Additional support from the mayors include holding the committee meetings in the mayor's conference room, provision of meals for committee meetings, office space for on-site Healthy Cities project staff and provision of financial support for the health/drug walk. One city committee was solicited by a United States congressman to help develop health care clinic for the poor and needy. A city councilman also serves as a member of this committee. A state legislator in one of the cities sponsored a resolution in support of promoting Healthy Cities in Indiana, and state legislators from each of the other five cities supported the resolution and it was passed by the Indiana General Assembly in 1990.

As a result of participation in Healthy Cities Indiana, what public policies have been changed and how have or will those changes impact upon the health of the community? Dye presents a useful definition of public policy that guides the discussion, 'public policy is whatever governments chose to do or not to do' (Dye 1972: 2). Using this definition, all cities have made active progress in promoting healthy public policies. Two small cities have taken steps to implement curbside recycling of solid-waste and one of the large cities is looking at reducing the solid waste stream. Another large city is developing an environmental policy plan for the city. Two cities have been working on developing an education programme for teen parents, one of these has obtained state funding for the programme, and the other local funding. Another small city has been working with state

Table 9.1 Healthy Cities action strategies

City	Short term	Long range
A	City-wide directory of services	Development of community-based substance abuse programme emphasizing self/community esteem
B	Healthy Cities poster contest in schools	Development of environmental 'master plan' for city
	Vision Workshops	Formation of youth Healthy Cities programme based in neighbourhoods
C	'Healthy Moments' radio public service announcements	Recreation programme for teens 15–18 years
	Recycling Day	Development of health programme to reduce high mortality rates
		Advocacy for 'healthful zoning' decisions
D	Family Walking Club	Development of central agency and facility for provision of emergency services
	Health fairs/Screenings	Development of assessment and referral programme for at-risk populations
	Mouthguard programme for youth	Everybody Wins programme to develop low income housing
	'Healthy Moments' radio public service announcements	Development of programme to assist at-risk youth
E	Family drug education event	Trash hauler, Crimewatch programme and safe-haven for children
	Neighbourhood directories of community services	In-school health and education programmes for teen parents
F	'Healthy Moments' radio public service announcements	School health/education programme for teen parents
	Health fairs for health education and screening	Development of indigent health care clinic
	Recycling packets for policy makers	Development of curbside recycling programme
	Recycling bins for drop-off recycling	Development of substance abuse programme

and national dental associations to increase the number of sports recommended for mouthguard protection.

In addition to these individual city examples, the resolution mentioned above and passed by the Indiana General Assembly in 1990 was developed and supported by the network of six Healthy Cities. Although the resolution does not carry any state fiscal responsibility, it was the first attempt by the cities to make a successful impact on state health policy, and one of the first formal acknowledgements of the state's responsibility for community health promotion.

Healthy Cities Indiana is being successfully implemented in all six cities. The smaller cities were able to initiate the Healthy Cities process at a faster rate than the larger cities. Although the complexity of community health problems did not vary across cities, the fact that in the larger cities more people were involved in the problems and the solutions delayed action. The network of community resources in smaller cities was more easily mobilized than in the larger cities. It was found that 'success breeds success', that is, local action empowers community leaders to take further action. In two large cities, the community resources were unknown to not only the Healthy Cities committee members, but also to service providers and local residents. These cities utilized the situation as an opportunity to identify their cities' strengths, and compiled community services directories for use by local people and agencies.

It also was found that committees that have too many professionals can delay local action. In part this is because professionals usually do not carry out the work that has been decided upon by the committees. Also, some health professionals and other community leaders were found to control committee action. If the committees were not broad-based or balanced enough, they had difficulty overcoming local vested interests. The Healthy Cities Indiana Committee Effectiveness Inventory was completed by members of the Healthy Cities committees and the results were used by the committees to expand their membership and form subcommittees or steering groups as mechanisms to carry out the work of the committees.

A basic set of Healthy Cities materials was needed and has been developed during the Healthy Cities Indiana project. These materials were not prepared at the outset of community leadership development in Healthy Cities, which would have enhanced community development. The network of Healthy Cities Indiana has facilitated community leadership development. It is during network sessions and other direct contact that community leaders learn from each other.

Based on the work in Healthy Cities Indiana, Indiana University School of Nursing Institute of Action Research for Community Health was designated as the WHO Collaborating Centre in Healthy Cities in January 1991. This centre is involved in continuing to identify research needs relevant to the Healthy Cities movement, conducting and collaborating in the planning and execution of qualitative and quantitative research in Healthy Cities and collaborating in the development of a global database in Healthy Cities. In addition, the centre is providing training opportunities for people interested in Healthy Cities, including community leaders, health professionals, scholars and fellows, visiting scientists and research trainees of WHO. The centre is also organizing and hosting national and international conferences on issues relevant to the Healthy Cities movement. Finally, the Centre issues periodic reports on the Healthy Cities movement and promotes information exchange about Healthy Cities programmes, research and resources.

Facilitative of Healthy Cities information exchange is the recent grant award from the W. K. Kellogg Foundation to disseminate the successful experiences of Healthy Cities Indiana. This grant supports the further development of Healthy Cities materials, including a Healthy Cities manual for community leaders and public health professionals, videotapes and workshop materials. A subcontract has been made with the National League of Cities which allows dissemination of Healthy Cities information through the National League of Cities Local Exchange Network, an electronic mail and on-line data base system, and through the *Nation's Cities Weekly* which has a circulation of 27,000. In addition, the WHO Collaborating Centre in Healthy Cities has developed a network of Healthy Cities worldwide, which also provides avenues for dissemination.

CONCLUSIONS: STRENGTH IN DIVERSITY

Consistent with American pluralism, there are a number of useful health promotion models in the United States that support communities as they address complex health problems at the local level. Unlike the European and Canadian experiences, Healthy Cities emerges in the United States not as one approach, but as diverse approaches with similar terminology which is confusing to community leaders and public health professionals. The National Consensus Conference on Efforts to Improve Public Health advanced the understanding of the various health promotion approaches and their contribution to achieving the national health objectives.

Each Healthy Cities or Healthy Communities approach to date originated independently and at different times, was based on different philosophical orientations and had different sponsoring organizations and funding. It is expected that the various types of Healthy Cities and health promotion efforts will continue to expand as cities request assistance from the different efforts underway.

There is wide diversity among cities in the United States. This diversity is not only because of geographic, economic, political and cultural differences, but also because the legal structure varies greatly from state to state. This diversity impacts on attempts to implement national programmes. Because of these factors, a centralized and co-ordinated health promotion or Healthy Cities movement is unlikely or inappropriate in the United States. In fact, to centralize this movement would hinder the development of community-based health promotion. Diverse communities need exposure to multiple health promotion models. Dissemination of these models through various mechanisms will continue to best support communities in their quest for improved community health.

ACKNOWLEDGEMENTS

The author wishes to express her appreciation to Melinda Rider, Associate Project Director, Healthy Cities Indiana for her thoughtful comments and suggestions on an early draft of this chapter.

Chapter 10

Building bridges between knowledge and action

The Canadian process of Healthy Communities indicators

Michel O'Neill

INTRODUCTION

Translating knowledge into practice is not easy. This chapter will expand the issue with reference to the development of indicators for the Healthy Communities project in Canada. An initiative of the Federal Ministry of Health and Welfare, known as Knowledge Development in Health Promotion, was born following the federal government's commitment to health promotion made in 1986 by the then minister, Jake Epp. It concerns the development and the dissemination of appropriate knowledge to undertake effective and meaningful health promotion interventions. In 1990–91, a major component of this initiative was to provide seed money for workshops held across the country; the theme suggested for these workshops was Indicators for Healthy Communities.

About 400 people of various backgrounds, all interested in building bridges between users and producers of knowledge in this context, were involved. The study of this series of events occurring around Healthy Cities (called hereafter Healthy Communities as is the custom in Canada) is of significant interest because Canada is often seen as an international leader in the field of health promotion. Analysing the process that took place there, in what can be seen as very good conditions, can thus shed some light on the possibilities and limits of the interaction between knowledge and practice in the context of the Healthy Cities movement and, more generally, in health promotion.

This chapter is divided into five sections. In the first two, background elements concerning the workshops, in the context of the Knowledge Development initiative and Healthy Communities project, are provided within the general framework of health promotion developments in Canada. The third section provides a description of the workshops series, whereas the fourth and the fifth analyse whether or not their objectives were met. Finally, the conclusion discusses more generally what has been learnt in this process in terms of the interaction between knowledge and practice.

THE KNOWLEDGE DEVELOPMENT IN HEALTH PROMOTION INITIATIVE

Canada has been heralded by many as a pioneer of health promotion (Kickbusch 1986; Green and Kreuter 1991). The first step in this pioneering role is usually identified as the Lalonde Report, *A New Perspective on the Health of Canadians* (Lalonde 1974). This report, mostly due to the thinking of a senior civil servant named Hubert Laframboise, has been acknowledged internationally for almost two decades as a landmark, by people as diverse as Illich (1975) and Green and Kreuter (1991).

The key element of the Lalonde Report was the fact that, for the first time, the national government of a major industrialized country endorsed the analyses of epidemiologists like McKeown (1976). For more than twenty years, they had argued that medical care was not the major factor in the decline of mortality rates observed over the past century in developed countries. Through the concept of the health field (Lalonde 1974), the report highlighted four major determinants of health: biology, environment, lifestyles and medical services. It went on to advocate further investment in the first three rather than the latter, the usual in advanced industrial societies.

The Lalonde Report has probably had more influence outside Canada than inside. In Canada, it has been severely criticized as an ideological framework to cut federal transfer payments to the provinces (Renaud 1981; Lesemann 1981) which, in Canada, are constitutionally responsible for the planning and provision of the health and welfare service. It was also accused of being a rhetorical exercise that was only partially enacted (Labonté and Penfold 1981; McEwen 1979; Ziglio 1988). It is nevertheless hard to deny the fact that this document was the first push on a wheel that was going to turn increasingly quickly as time went on.

One of the effects of the report was the creation, at the end of the 1970s, of the first Health Promotion Directorate in the federal government of an industrialized country. It was where spontaneously, at the beginning of the 1980s, representatives of the European Region of the World Health Organisation (WHO) sought advice in revising their health education programme in the context of WHO's Health for All strategy (Kickbusch 1986). These consultations were so fruitful during the first half of the 1980s that, from this relationship between Health and Welfare Canada and WHO/Euro, the field of health promotion developed its high visibility.

The links between WHO and Canada in the international diffusion of health promotion were demonstrated in the First International Conference on Health Promotion held in Ottawa in November 1986. Co-sponsored by WHO and Health and Welfare Canada, jointly with the Canadian Public Health Association, the conference produced the Ottawa Charter for Health Promotion (WHO 1986) which has since been translated into about twenty languages and which is generally considered as proposing the most widely accepted definition of the concept of health promotion.

The Ottawa Conference was the outcome of a significant internal process within Health and Welfare Canada whereby, from 1985 onwards, the production of a national health policy document based on the principles of health promotion was undertaken. This process led to the first important declaration by the then Minister of Health and Welfare, Jake Epp, in June 1986 (Epp 1986a). This was followed by another famous document, 'Achieving Health for All: A Framework for Health Promotion' (Epp 1986b), released in November 1986, at the end of the Ottawa Conference. Finally, this document was not a formal statement of policy, but rather a discussion paper to generate debate about the ways in which health should be pursued in Canada. The Epp framework was seen by many as innovative, if somewhat unclear and confused, because of the fact that it brought onto the political agenda ideas like reduction in inequalities and fostering community participation. However, it must be remembered that the Epp document was released by a conservative government at a time when the strength of the neo-conservative ideology and the fiscal crisis of the federal government in Canada had created structural conditions unfavourable to the implementation of such policy (O'Neill 1989). This had not been the case when the Lalonde Report was published. The appearance of such a document was thus not a guarantee that health promotion would in practice move up the agenda of the federal government, a government which, in any case, has no constitutional right to intervene in health services.

Several processes were nevertheless undertaken by the federal bureaucracy following the appearance of the Epp document. These processes continued even after the replacement of Epp by two other ministers. Some of these developments led to a widespread consultation on the Epp framework in Canada, to the funding from 1988 to 1991 of two major national programmes (Healthy Communities and Strengthening Community Health) as well as to the launch of the Knowledge Development initiative. It is this latter initiative that will be explored further in this chapter because of its particular orientation concerning linkages between research and practice and, more specifically, because of its application to indicators for Healthy Communities.

As described in three key documents (Rootman 1988; Rootman 1989; Health and Welfare Canada 1990), the general purpose of this initiative was to meet the challenge of translating the key concepts of the Epp framework into action. Figure 10.1 shows these concepts within this general framework.

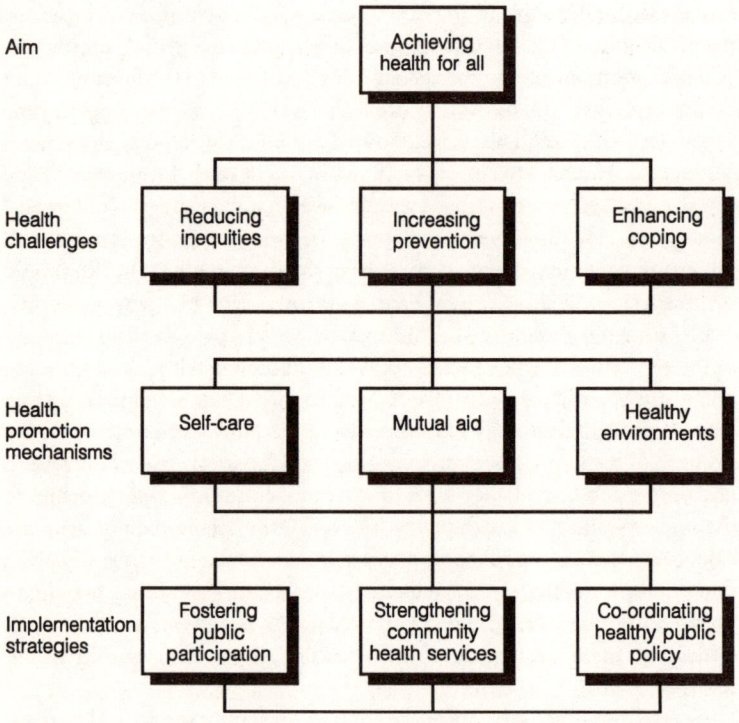

Figure 10.1 A framework for health promotion
Source: Epp (1986b: 8)

Moreover, by shifting the focus from an individual to a broader environmental perspective, the framework invites the involvement of disciplines, sectors and interests which previously had not necessarily considered health part of their domain. 'Research will have a vital role to play in establishing and legitimizing the health promotion approach presented in achieving Health for All' (Health and Welfare Canada 1990: 4).

The general vision of the initiative was not just to produce academic research through new types of disciplinary or interdisciplinary endeavours. It also sought to draw on the knowledge developed in service agencies or in grass-roots organizations, and to insist on the circulation and diffusion of all these types of knowledge. Consequently, the general title of this initiative is not Research Development but Knowledge Development. In order to sensitize academics and other researchers to this vision of knowledge as well as to develop priorities for funding and development, a thorough and sophisticated process was proposed.

To begin with, two working groups of experts, one internal to Health and Welfare and one external, were convened in 1987 to 'recommend priority areas and strategies for research' (Health and Welfare Canada 1990: 5). In order to assist these working groups, a series of literature reviews was commissioned on topics directly related to the framework (Rootman 1989), some of which have become internationally well known (Pederson *et al.* 1988). Out of these literature reviews and out of the final report of the two working groups, a final draft discussion paper entitled 'Priorities and Strategies for Research to Promote the Health of Canadians' was prepared during the spring of 1988. It was the end of what could be called the problem-definition phase of the initiative.

The second phase, the consultation, was conducted between September 1988 and May 1989. It involved the presentation of the draft discussion paper in thirty-two workshops organized all over the country. These workshops involved more than 1,000 people from a wide range of fields and disciplines, including health practitioners, academic researchers and bureaucrats, producers and users of knowledge for health promotion. The output of all these local workshops was eventually discussed at a national workshop held in Ottawa in May of 1989, and a final report was then submitted to Health and Welfare Canada.

The third phase, which has been called the action phase of the initiative (Health and Welfare Canada 1990: 12), began in the autumn of 1989. It involved the creation of a National Advisory Committee on Health Promotion Research, whose function 'was to provide the Health Services and Health Promotion branch with guidance and assistance, to carry out a variety of lobbying and advocacy tasks, to raise awareness and interest at the community and regional levels and to relay the views of people on the ground to the Federal Government' (Health and Welfare Canada, 1990:

12). Since the beginning of this phase, several important actions have been undertaken, under the guidance of the Advisory Committee.

A special competition to secure finance for health promotion research was held in 1989, in order to stimulate the presentation of projects on this topic to the National Health Research and Development Programme (NHRDP). This is one of the major funding sources for academic research in the health sector in Canada. Moreover, the first joint venture ever undertaken by NHRDP and the Social Sciences and Humanities Research Council was prompted by the Knowledge Development initiative. Announced in early 1991, this special programme will provide seed money to the amount of Can. $500,000 a year for five years, to six centres for health promotion research across Canada, an investment of Can. $3.0 million.

A synthesis of the literature reviews which had been commissioned by Health and Welfare Canada was prepared and widely distributed (Health and Welfare Canada 1989). A *Knowledge Development Newsletter*, purporting to reinforce and expand the network of people interested in knowledge development was begun. By the end of 1991, two issues had been published. A national list of health promotion researchers was also produced and distributed, with annual updates. Finally, the first national conference on health promotion research entitled 'Health Promotion Research Methods: Expanding the Repertoire', was held in Toronto in early December 1990, drawing over 400 people from all over Canada. A selection of some of the key papers of this conference are in the *Canadian Journal of Public Health*, Supplement 1 to Volume 83, 1992.

However, probably the most visible part of the action phase of the Knowledge Development initiative in 1990–91 was the organization of the already mentioned series of workshops on indicators for Healthy Communities.

ANALYSING THE WORKSHOPS ON INDICATORS FOR HEALTHY COMMUNITIES: SOME CONTEXTUAL ELEMENTS

The idea of holding a series of workshops in the context of the Knowledge Development initiative was linked to two needs which emerged from the consultation phase of this initiative. First, the need to create, or support and enlarge, regional networks of people interested in knowledge for health promotion practice; and second, the need to fund directed research that contributes to the health promotion knowledge base. In order to have some guidance about the ways in which to fulfil these needs, a preliminary national workshop involving about twenty people from across the country was convened in Ottawa in December 1989, on the topic of indicators to measure health promotion. This topic was selected because in the consultation phase it had frequently emerged as a top priority and because of the work already begun on this issue by a group in the Prairies region.

The day was divided into two parts. First, Horst Noak from the University of Berne in Switzerland, a health promotion researcher well known for his work on indicators, presented his view of the issues. Second, the participants in working groups tried to discuss how a national endeavour on this topic could be developed. At the end of this workshop there was agreement that:

1 the topic was too complex to be addressed in general;
2 focusing the indicators discussion on a precise area was much more likely to yield some kind of result in a single year span;
3 the Healthy Communities project, in which there was a pressing need for reflection on indicators and evaluation as well as for a series of indicators to be used by the municipalities across the country, should be the focus as the Prairies group had already chosen; and
4 regional workshops should be funded for this purpose, encouraging but not forcing them to work on this topic, given the variations in regional dynamics.

The person in charge of the initiative in Ottawa thus approached people in the five national regions as defined by Health and Welfare Canada: the Pacific region (British Columbia, Alberta and Yukon), the Prairies region (Saskatchewan, Manitoba and the North-West Territories), Ontario region, Quebec region, and Atlantic region (New Brunswick, Nova Scotia, Newfoundland and Prince Edward Island). He provided for each one, through the Health and Welfare Canada Regional Health Promotion Office, a sum of Can. $8,000 as seed money to organize the workshop. The overall goal of this workshop was twofold. First, to encourage the development of a regional network of people interested in health promotion knowledge by building bridges between various academic disciplines, between academic people and various agencies, and between users and producers of knowledge; and second, to try to create an evolutionary process whereby the knowledge of indicators for Healthy Communities developed in one regional workshop could be used by the other workshops and integrated, at the end of the year, in a national body of knowledge that could then be disseminated.

The birth of the international Healthy Cities movement occurred in Canada in 1984, in the wake of a conference entitled Healthy Toronto

2000: Beyond Health Care (Canadian Journal of Public Health 1985). It was there that the two originators of the concept, Leonard Duhl of Berkeley, California and Trevor Hancock of Toronto, as well as its facilitator, Ilona Kickbusch from WHO in Copenhagen, began to see the potential of the idea. However, it was not in North America that the Healthy Cities movement first got off the ground. It began in 1986 as a small project in the European region of WHO/Euro (WHO Healthy Cities Project 1988b) purporting to implement the Health for All and health promotion visions developed over the first half of the decade by the WHO health education team in Copenhagen. However, it began to gather so much interest that it was soon to be transformed, in Europe and elsewhere afterwards, as 'the project that became a movement' (Tsouros 1990b).

The international history of the movement is now well known and has started to be studied more thoroughly (Tsouros 1990b; Curtice and McQueen 1990; O'Neill *et al.* 1990; Baum and Brown 1989; Fortin *et al.* 1991; De Leeuw 1990; Flynn and Rider 1991; Flynn *et al.* 1991; Ashton 1992). Wherever it develops, the Healthy Cities movement is basically about changing municipal policies in order to create a health-enhancing environment (Hancock and Duhl 1986).

In Canada, because of the development of the European project with which Trevor Hancock was associated, due to the Ottawa Conference on Health Promotion where the European Healthy Cities project was presented, and with the return to Canada at about the same time of people who had studied in Berkeley with Leonard Duhl, the first national group of interested people began to coalesce in 1986. The first city to formally become a healthy community was Rouyn-Noranda in April 1987, because of the leadership of another key player on the Canadian scene: Réal Lacombe. With some help from the Canadian Public Health Association, and with the co-sponsorship of the Canadian Institute of Planners and the Canadian Association of Municipalities, a Can. $680,000 proposal for a three-year grant was submitted to Health and Welfare Canada and was funded from 1 April 1988 to 31 March 1991. This allowed for a national secretariat to be developed in order to stimulate the development of the movement.

The patterns of development in Quebec and in the rest of Canada were very different though. In Quebec, under the leadership of community health professionals, a strong network called *Villes et villages en santé* took off quite quickly and effectively without much help from the national secretariat, with a Centre of Promotion and Information located in Quebec City playing a major networking function. The Quebec network included in the middle of 1992 seventy-five cities and villages (O'Neill *et al*. 1990; Fortin *et al*. 1991). In the rest of the country, individual cities here and there joined, but it is only recently that another province, British Columbia, invested significant amounts of money and got its network going. These provincial (or regional in certain cases) networks are now the privileged development tool of the movement because the funding of a national secretariat was not renewed after April 1991. According to the Director of the Canadian Institute of Planning (Sherwood 1991), it is hard to accurately estimate the number of Canadian communities which have formally joined the movement; a total of about 160, including the seventy-five from Quebec, was the estimate given in June 1992. That many of these communities expressed the need to obtain indicators to evaluate their process was another reason why the Knowledge Development initiative decided to prioritize this topic for its series of workshops.

The analysis of this series of workshops presented in this chapter was conducted using the following data.

1 *Participant observation* The author was personally involved in the series in four ways: as a member of the advisory committee which decided to implement the workshops; as a participant in the three national workshops held about indicators (the preliminary one held in Ottawa in December 1989 and the two held in Toronto in November 1990, in the context of the First National Conference on Health Promotion Research); as a participant in the workshop steering committee that met three times, which was a loose structure including the organizers of the six regional workshops plus a few key civil servants of Health and Welfare Canada and, in some instances, organizers of the regional workshops; and as a participant in three of the five regional workshops that were finally held.

2 *Documentation* In addition to the proceedings of the regional workshops (Feather and Mathur 1990; Craig *et al*. 1991; O'Neill and Cardinal 1992), the author had access to a wide variety of unpublished documents (minutes of meetings, programmes and lists of participants for the regional workshops, etc.). The quantity of these items varied depending on the amount of energy devoted to the process by the organizers of each regional workshop and on the degree of formality of the organization; not every organizing committee kept written records, for example.

3 *Questionnaire* A three-page questionnaire was sent in May 1991 to the six main organizers of the regional workshops in order to gather a

minimum of standardized information on each of them. The response
rate was 100 per cent.
4   *Personal communications*   Finally, a series of telephone calls was made in
November 1991 to clarify specific details with either some of the
workshop organizers or some of the Health and Welfare Canada civil
servants who were members of the steering committee.

A DESCRIPTION OF THE WORKSHOPS ON
INDICATORS FOR HEALTHY COMMUNITIES

This section provides descriptive information on the three national and on
the five regional workshops that were held during 1990–91 in the context
of the Knowledge Development initiative.

As described above, three national workshops occurred in relation to
the regional workshops process. The first one, held in Ottawa in December
1989, has already been mentioned. It served as the trigger mechanism to
focus the regional workshops on Indicators for Healthy Communities. The
two others were held in early December 1990, during the first national
conference on Health Promotion Research held in Toronto. Both sessions
were included in the regular programme as concurrent sessions and were
designed in the same manner. They lasted one and a half hours, and during
the first part the national co-ordinator of the initiative in Ottawa as well
as the co-ordinators of the six regional workshops presented progress
reports on the evolution of the process in their environment. The second
part was devoted to exchanges with the participants. At that point three
regional workshops had already been held (the Prairies one in Winnipeg,
the Pacific one in Vancouver and the Quebec one in Montreal) and three
were still in the planning process (the Ontarian one in Toronto, an
additional one in the Pacific region in Calgary and the Maritimes one).

The original intent of these transnational workshops in Toronto was
twofold. On the one hand, it was to offer to the researchers who had not
come to the regional workshops, which were by invitation, the opportunity to gain a sense of how the action phase of the Knowledge
Development initiative was unfolding in 1990–1. It was also to see whether
or not lessons could be drawn from the regional workshops process at about
mid-point in its development. Both workshops were well attended,
drawing an average of about thirty participants each, and were the occasion
of interesting and lively debates about Knowledge Development for health
promotion in general, and more specifically for Healthy Communities
indicators.

As for the six regional workshops, five of them were finally held. The

Maritimes workshop did not take place despite the efforts of the person who had accepted the organizational responsibility. Four out of these five workshops focused on data or indicators to evaluate Healthy Communities, whereas the Calgary one addressed the more general issue of the inclusion of health promotion in the Albertan health system. Except for the Ontarian workshop, which lasted one and a half days, these regional events each lasted one day.

Table 10.1 summarizes the type and amount of resources involved in the organization of the workshops.

Table 10.1   Resources involved in the organization of workshops on Healthy Communities indicators

	Number of agencies putting hard money in the workshop	Number of other agencies sponsoring and/or putting in-kind resources for the workshop	Total number of agencies involved	Total amount of hard money involved
Winnipeg	1	2	3	$8,000*
Vancouver	3	2	5	$20,000
Montreal	1	3	4	$8,000
Toronto	2	6	8	$18,000
Calgary	1	4	5	$8,000*
Total	8	17	25	$62,000

Note: *In these two cases, no amount being precisely reported, it is assumed that the minimal amount provided by Health and Welfare Canada was utilized.

In addition to what was provided by the Regional Health Promotion Offices of Health and Welfare Canada, all the workshops were either sponsored or were provided with resources in kind by a number of other agencies. In two cases the Offices of Health Promotion of provincial Ministries of Health, and in another a provincial Public Health Association allocated financial resources. The sponsorship or provision of resources in kind came mostly from academic sources as well as from a variety of provincial, regional or municipal health related agencies.

The leadership in the workshop organization was assumed by academics in three cases out of five, by a provincial non-governmental organization in one case and by a municipal department of health in the last. In all cases the organizing dynamics were the result of interactive processes between various organizations, linked to regional idiosyncrasies. This in itself can be seen as an interesting achievement.

WERE KNOWLEDGE BRIDGES BUILT BETWEEN VARIOUS DISCIPLINES AND CONSTITUENCIES?

In this section the outcome of the regional workshops will be analysed in relation to the first objective of the series by exploring if these five events contributed to fostering a relationship between various people interested in knowledge development for health promotion. First, the workshops' capacity to improve contacts among academic disciplines, especially among those not traditionally interested in health, will be reviewed. Second, whether academic researchers, as well as other constituencies, were able to build new bridges during these events will be investigated.

Before addressing the outcome of the bridge-building process, it is interesting to note that the 273 people who attended the five workshops constitute 76 per cent of the people who had been invited. The invitational status of the process (basically determined by the amount of money available, which hardly allowed the organization of open meetings) gave a useful margin of manoeuvre to the organizers who could fine-tune this list according to the specific objectives of their activity. At the same time it created some unease in certain areas because of the expectations raised with at least 1,000 people during the consultation phase of the initiative.

As can be seen in Table 10.2, the two most prevalent categories of attenders were people from local or regional health units (25 per cent of total participants) as well as academics (24 per cent). Three other groups participated at about the same rate: community representatives (12 per cent), civil servants coming from municipal governments (11 per cent) as well as provincial civil servants (11 per cent). Federal civil servants of the Health Promotion Branch of Health and Welfare Canada (be it from Ottawa or from regional offices) were also constant around 6 per cent, but the politicians were much less visible, only eight coming from municipal governments (3 per cent) and none from the provincial level. The final category 'Others' (7 per cent) includes a variety of people.

Academics were one of the most numerous subgroups attending the workshops. Moreover, as was also indicated in Table 10.2, each workshop attracted people from a variety of disciplines. In the questionnaire, the organizers were asked to name the major disciplines of the academics invited. The list revealed that nine different social or behavioural sciences were mentioned (behavioural science, education, geography, political science, psychology, public administration, regional planning, social work, sociology), eight health sciences (community or public health, geronto- logy, health sciences, medicine, nursing, physical education, rehabilitation

Table 10.2 Distribution of regional workshop participants according to type of milieu

Workshop	Academics	Federal civil servants	Provincial civil servants	Municipal civil servants	Provincial politicians	Municipal politicians	Regional or local workers in health agencies	Community represen- tatives	Others	Total
Winnipeg	23 (10)*	6	5	1	0	0	6	1	1	43 (15.7%)
Vancouver	17 (8)*	3	7	11	0	4	19	11	0	72 (26.4%)
Montreal	4 (3)*	2	1	6	0	1	18	0	4	36 (13.2%)
Toronto	12 (10)*	4	6	8	0	3	20	13	15	81 (29.7%)
Calgary	10 (5)*	2	10	5	0	0	5	9	0	41 (15.0%)
Total	66 (24.2%)	17 (6.2%)	29 (10.6%)	31 (11.4%)	0 (0%)	8 (3.0%)	68 (24.9%)	34 (12.4%)	20 (7.3%)	273 (100%)

Note: *Number of different disciplines represented
Source: Questionnaire sent to workshop organizers

medicine, social and preventive medicine), as well as one natural science (biology).

Does this mean that individuals or disciplines new to the field of health promotion were attracted by the workshops? First, there were significant variations between the workshops as to their willingness, and their success, in bringing in new and diverse academics. In Winnipeg, where the focus of the workshop was specifically on the academic clientele, it is obvious from the proceedings (Feather and Mathur 1990) that attracting new and diverse people worked well because it was the main focus of the workshop. In Montreal, however, the focus was more on offering the non-academic researchers, who had already begun to deal with the practicalities of evaluating Healthy Communities projects at the local level, the opportunity to get input from a variety of academic as well as non-academic resources. Attracting new and diverse academics was a total failure despite the number of invitations made to this clientele. Moreover, despite a fair number and variety of academics at the Vancouver workshop, this meeting gave more the impression of individuals already interested, if not involved, in health promotion research who used the occasion to get together, rather than the inclusion of people totally new to the field who were brought there to explore new avenues together, as was the case in Winnipeg.

Academics are not necessarily willing to get involved in things that do not seem directly related to their very specific interests. Attracting them to Healthy Cities or health promotion research is not necessarily an easy task, especially if the focus of Knowledge Development is not academic research. It seems, however, that it is not an impossible task, as shown, among other things, by a process undertaken by the Ontario Prevention Clearinghouse before the Knowledge Development workshops, whereby hundreds of Ontario researchers were invited to eight workshops (Stirling 1991). Academics, especially if they have not previously been involved in what they see as health-related matters, will thus be very cautious to see how the new ventures suggested by health promotion meet their very narrow and specific interests.

To pursue a little further the discussion on the involvement of new types of academics in health promotion knowledge development, the Winnipeg workshop will be examined in detail for two reasons. First, it is the only place where several specific objectives of the workshop were primarily targeted to the development of new links between academics of various universities and disciplines, in order, among other things, to pursue the creation of a Prairies network of health promotion researchers. Second, the written material about this specific workshop is detailed and includes a retrospective analysis of the process by the organizers (Feather and Mathur 1990; Feather 1990).

For the Winnipeg conference organizers, several things constrained the creation of new interdisciplinary exchanges over health promotion and Healthy Communities indicators. First, the fact that the Prairies region of Health and Welfare Canada (two provinces and one territory) is a meaningless, artificially created region caused an additional complication in trying to link academics (Feather 1990: 1). This problem has also been mentioned in some form or other by the two other regions (Pacific and Maritimes) which, unlike Ontario and Quebec where one province equals one region, are a combination of several provinces or territories.

A second difficulty in the Prairies region was the paucity of past collaboration between universities in health promotion matters (Feather 1990: 1). In addition, during the workshop, two further problems emerged (Feather and Mathur 1990: 21–32). Despite the interest and even the enthusiasm of some people for the opportunity to interact, there were extreme difficulties in finding a common scientific ground. This was due to basic differences in concept definition, in epistemological positions or in research methods that showed most vividly when the various subgroups undertook the task of agreeing on a list of indicators. There was also considerable scepticism from the academics who pointed out that the federal government was sending a double message by encouraging people to go for interdisciplinary ventures but, at the same time, cutting back on general research funding and not providing specific funding sources allowing the kind of research required for health promotion.

The difficulties of apparent agreement over concepts (Feather 1990: 5) and of reconciliation between divergent epistemological paradigms were also highlighted in the Vancouver workshop (Hayes 1991). Thus it seems that the workshops succeeded more in showing the significant barriers to interdisciplinary academic work than in building new interdisciplinary bridges. The process of developing interdisciplinary academic work is of the same nature and as difficult as the intersectoral process requested of communities by the health promotion rhetoric (O'Neill 1990: 36). Indeed, the rewards systems and promotion mechanisms of academics (disciplinary structure of departments, disciplinary publication requirements, lack of flexibility in accounting mechanisms of universities and of funding agencies for inter-departmental or inter-university research) are structurally organized in such a way as to almost preclude any kind of interdisciplinary exchanges in the same way that bureaucratic segmentation of agencies makes it very difficult to work intersectorally.

Hence, the workshops revealed that if they were seen as part of an ongoing process rather than as a one-off enterprise they could probably be useful in helping to alleviate the important barriers already mentioned. However, it was also pointed out that altering the structural environment by manipulating the criteria and ways in which research money is allocated could have a much more important effect because 'researchers will go where the money is' (Feather 1990: 6).

If building interdisciplinary bridges among academics of various sorts was not really achieved in the workshops, were the bridges between academics and non-academics any easier to build? The suspicion is that it depends very much on how the invitations to the workshops were made. Having had the privilege to participate in several of them, it is obvious that the more diversified the groups invited, the bigger the clash between various cultures pertaining to knowledge and its utilization. Even if academics can argue about almost everything, they will usually agree on the fact that science and rigour are important in knowledge production as well as on the conviction that academics are the ones best trained to do science properly. The clash is thus very important when politicians claim that they do not really care about science if they get the information that can make them look good in the press in order to help their chances of re-election, when bureaucrats want administrative information to monitor programmes and allocate resources immediately and when community groups want to hear success stories about things that worked elsewhere in order to replicate them right away. The meaning of 'knowledge' for health promotion practice can thus be far removed from the usual scientific vision of it held by academics.

This might sound somewhat like a caricature. However, among the various constituencies which have a stake in health promotion in general, or, more specifically, in a project such as Healthy Communities, academics are but one group. Academics had to negotiate their legitimacy and usefulness in the various workshops attended. The fiercest debates were usually between local politicians and academics; the former were usually less impressed than community representatives by the prestige and status of academics. Politicians are also used to arguing, cajoling, negotiating and insisting on the immediate usefulness of information.

This does not mean that the workshops were places where people from these various constituencies could not learn from each other or begin to find out about the usefulness of the other group's perspective. Given their invitation strategy, the Vancouver and Toronto workshops actually seem to have succeeded in gathering a variety of people who were already interested in some way in the utilization of knowledge to aid Healthier Communities. It was as if these two workshops acted as catalysts to show people that, despite their differences, they share the same basic ideology, can find a way to work out their different views and can find a complementarity between their various skills.

There is no simple straightforward solution to the production and dissemination of knowledge between the various constituencies interested in health promotion activities. Academics are only one group with specific skills that can contribute to the overall effort – a position which is very unusual and uncomfortable for many of them.

WHAT WAS LEARNT ABOUT THE UTILIZATION OF INDICATORS FOR HEALTHY COMMUNITIES?

As described above, the second goal of the workshops was to generate knowledge about indicators for Healthy Communities. Were they successful in achieving this goal? The mechanisms through which learning was to occur were not clearly specified at the outset of the process. Consequently, no systematic plan was made about publications nor about the sharing of the information gained in one workshop with the participants of other workshops or with other people, be they researchers or not. The only informal mechanism that was put in place was the workshop's steering committee already alluded to, which, among other things, allowed the organizers of individual workshops to attend some of the other workshops.

The National Advisory Committee on Health Promotion Research, which is a more formal body than the workshops' steering committee, followed up the whole process at a certain distance but did not perceive its role as dealing with the mechanics of workshop organization. Moreover, during the year when the workshops occurred, the person who had been responsible for the Knowledge Development initiative resigned from Health and Welfare and was successively replaced by three other people who did not have the time or the knowledge of the initiative to ensure its evolution at the pace it could have maintained otherwise. This lack of stability played a major part in the absence of precise mechanisms that would have helped to ensure better accumulation of knowledge developed from the workshops. More attention should thus be paid to this issue in future similar initiatives lest an important objective of the whole venture be missed. Despite this lack of a formal mechanism to integrate what happened, there are several lessons which can be drawn from the workshops on the topic of indicators.

The primary, and probably most important, lesson is the fact that there is no magic list of indicators that can be universally utilized. This might appear to be an obvious statement but, before the workshops, the hope that a standardised set of valid and reliable indicators for Healthy Communities would emerge as an outcome of the process was anticipated. There appear to be a number of reasons why this did not happen.

First, due to the scope of the concepts used by the Healthy Cities movement, literally thousands of indicators of all kinds are available to measure almost any dimension of any of these concepts. Cardinal and O'Neill (1992) review a series of indicators lists which have been specifically developed all over the world for Healthy Cities or Healthy Communities projects and which vary dramatically in terms of their scope, as well as in the number of indicators included. Second, indicators or related data can be used for one or more purposes, for example the production of scientific information; the monitoring of the evolution of the local project; comparisons with other cities or villages; the renewal of funding for the project and so on. Third, information can be collected to assess various things, including the health status of a municipality; the process of introducing Healthy Communities into a municipality; and the impact of such development. Fourth, the results may be dramatically different depending on who requests the information or indicators to be collected and on who paid for such a collection and who uses it.

Another major lesson is that addressing the issue of indicators or information to build healthier communities is always a complicated, if not a conflictual process. This is due mainly to the fact that everywhere, several groups or individuals, having different visions of the world and different power to impose it on others, will suggest different ways to evaluate Healthy Communities projects. This is almost inescapable in a movement like Healthy Cities where, due to the intersectoral and the participative dimensions of the concept, many players are inevitably brought into the game.

There is no single and easy way to resolve the conflicts that will almost inevitably occur, but knowing that they are likely to happen diminishes their negative effect. This leads us to the final important lesson drawn from the workshops. It is absolutely necessary for any Healthy Communities project, whatever the level it operates at (village, city, metropolis, national network of Healthy Communities or international), to make choices about the information or the indicators needed in its own specific case. The strategy to make these choices, and the outcome of the strategy, will necessarily depend on the political dynamics that will occur in a specific instance. It is our conclusion that there is no better way to make these choices, and that, as pointed out especially in the Toronto regional workshop, the very process of deciding on which kind of information or indicators to use is in itself a key element, almost regardless of the result of this process.

These lessons may seem unpleasant to those who would dream of standardized measurements, of comparability between communities who have joined the Healthy Cities movement and communities who have not, and of other rigorous evaluations. These things might eventually be achieved in the form of academic research projects, but as long as the focus is the real life of a city project, it seems to us that pragmatism is the order of the day, and that it takes a certain degree of advancement of the local projects before evaluation, information and indicators begin to be an issue at all (Stirling 1991).

All these conclusions might seem self-evident, simplistic or not technical enough. They are, however, the most important outcome of the work-shops, alerting everybody interested in these issues to the fact that the business of developing indicators or information to build healthier com-munities is more than anything else a political process, not a technical one.

CONCLUSION: FINAL COMMENTS ABOUT THE LINKS BETWEEN KNOWLEDGE AND PRACTICE IN HEALTH PROMOTION

A first major analytical clue about the evolution of the Canadian Knowl-edge Development initiative in health promotion emerges from the discussions conducted up to now. Especially for non-Canadians who generally tend to associate the Canadian achievements in health promotion with the federal government, our analyses show the real dynamics of Canadian federal–provincial relationships when an area of provincial jurisdiction is at stake. Thus, it is not because the federal government has the willingness or even money to spend that, automatically, regions or provinces follow. In the specific case of the workshops, one of the regions (the Pacific) held two workshops instead of one because of the idiosyn-crasies of subregional dynamics; one workshop was not held (the Maritimes one) and one workshop was not on the suggested theme (the Calgary one).

Nevertheless, in four instances out of a possible six, information for Healthy Communities was the key theme, even if the approach to treating it varied to take into account the various provincial or regional situations. It thus shows that, overall, federal discourse and money have indeed a country-wide effect on the evolution of provincial or regional issues, even in matters (like health services or health promotion) where, in theory, the federal government should not be involved because they constitutionally belong to the provinces. However, the workshops show that this effect is strongly mediated by the provincial and regional circumstances, a point that should be carefully remembered by non-Canadians looking at what is going on in Canada.

Another important point to remember in the kind of venture like the workshops is the risk of lack of follow-up. In Ottawa, the Knowledge Development for health promotion was never a real programme inserted in the bureaucratic machinery of yearly budgets, but rather an initiative largely dependent upon the people who cared for it. This leaves it very vulnerable. In spite of all that has been achieved over the past years, it takes time and energy to make sure that the newsletter continues to be published, that a process to collectivize and disseminate the knowledge gathered in the workshops is set up, that a strategic plan for the years to come is designed and that the initiatives undertaken to fund health promotion research are maintained and operate well.

Despite the dedication of the various people who replaced one another as project officers of the initiative, there is a constant fear that the whole thing will fail. Years of efforts and commitments might very well get lost in the vagaries of political and bureaucratic changes and the major efforts invested to encourage the very difficult task to build bridges between various types of knowledge producers and users of health promotion might be wasted. Due to its marginality, both from a classical academic perspective and from a bureaucratic perspective, the initiative is thus quite fragile.

The difficulty of maintaining continuity and developing a strong network of health promotion knowledge developers and users at the regional level was also pointed out specifically by three of the workshop organizers. The artificiality of Health and Welfare Canada's division of the country into regions is surely one of the problems. It is to alleviate such problems that the creation of a network of Centres for Health Promotion Research has been announced. The danger that these centres will only do research by academic rules and get disconnected from Knowledge Development, which is defined by a tension between several types of rules (especially the academic, the bureaucratic, the political and the community ones, as seen in the case of the workshops), is significant. The structure of the reward system related to these centres should thus include ways to force them to be run by a board where interests other than the academic are well represented, if not dominant, and ways to make sure that the research programme is both scientifically sound and relevant to the community.

Socially, academics are used to defining and dominating knowledge development. Health promotion invites them to play a different role, where they have to relinquish power but at the same time where they get the satisfaction of social relevance and usefulness. This is a kind of programme which is very hard to achieve, due to the structural constraints of the academic world. As has been shown in this chapter, it is not a totally impossible dream and an area like Healthy Communities is especially conducive to this type of evolution. We have also realized, however, that the road is rough and that only efforts lasting for a certain period in time will allow local, provincial, regional, national and international networks of various academics and non-academics to develop. The Knowledge Development initiative has been a key instrument to do just this in Canada.

ACKNOWLEDGEMENTS

The author wishes to thank the people successively in charge of the Knowledge Development initiative in the Health Promotion Directorate of Health and Welfare Canada in Ottawa, namely, Irving Rootman, Michael Nelson, Prudence Ford and especially Sylvain Paradis, who strongly supported the preparation of this chapter. He also wishes to acknowledge the collaboration of the various individuals who provided additional information on their workshop, namely, Joan Feather for the Prairies workshop, Sharon Manson-Singer for the Pacific one in Vancouver, Allison Stirling for the Ontarian one, Thomas Abernathy for Calgary as well as Dale Poel for the Maritimes. This chapter builds on the collective process of organizing these workshops; however, it presents a personal analysis that does not necessarily reflect the perspective of Health and Welfare Canada, nor of any of the people who provided information or feedback on earlier versions of this chapter. Many thanks as well to Mike Kelly, who converted into readable English a paper written with a heavy French accent!

Chapter 11

Evaluating the Healthy Cities Project in Drumchapel, Glasgow

Sarah McGhee and James McEwen

INTRODUCTION

This chapter describes the initial evaluation of the Drumchapel Healthy Cities Project set up in July 1990. Its purpose was to examine and confront health issues in Drumchapel, a post-war housing scheme in Glasgow with a population of around 22,000. Funding for the project came from the regional and district councils, the local health board and an intersectoral initiative which was already tackling social and economic issues in the area. The Initiative had been formed through partnership between the regional and district councils and the local community. The pilot project itself was resourced with a health promotion officer as co-ordinator, a resource and development worker, an administrative assistant, an office in a local community centre and a small budget for running expenses.

The project's executive group comprised representatives of the funding bodies (regional and district councils, Glasgow Healthy Cities Project and the local health board), the project co-ordinator, representatives from the local community organizations council and, eventually, a community health volunteer. The working group grew as the project developed and eventually comprised the project co-ordinator and resource and development worker; representatives of the community education, adult education and social work departments; local health visitors; a representative of the local volunteer project and several of the project's community health volunteers.

The executive and working groups were anxious that evaluation should proceed throughout the pilot phase and the Professor of Public Health at the local university (one of the representatives of the Healthy Cities project on the executive group) offered to collaborate in this. The academic department of Public Health provided a part-time researcher. This chapter will describe the approach to evaluation and how it proceeded throughout the first year of the project (rather than concentrating on details of results). But first the project itself is briefly described.

The project's overall philosophy was in line with the World Health Organization's aims of reducing inequalities in health, enabling people to reach more of their physical and mental potential, achieving community participation in health issues and co-operation between all local groups and agencies who can contribute to better health. To achieve these aims, the specific objectives for the first year were to establish executive and working groups, to develop ways of addressing the health issues identified by the local population in a Community Health Profile survey which had been recently conducted in the district, to draw up and implement a health strategy for the area, to mobilize, train and resource a network of community health volunteers, to establish a training programme and a health information and advice service for local residents and workers, to increase access to and encourage the provision of health counselling, self-help and support groups and to ensure adequate recording and evaluation of the work of the project.

Before the formal evaluation began, project staff had carried out a survey among local people to find out what information they would like to have available. The Health Resource Library was then stocked with books, leaflets and audiovisual material both for the use of the community and of local health workers. Later, personal advice sessions were offered three days a week with a health visitor and a mental health officer available on one afternoon every week.

THE EVALUATION

In determining which of the many aspects of the project to evaluate and the methods to use, the researchers took several factors into consideration. First, methods for the evaluation of health promotion projects such as this are not yet very well developed and examples are scarce in the literature, particularly for the evaluation of community health volunteering which was a novel aspect of this project. Second, there were differing viewpoints on the purpose of the evaluation and hence on the appropriate approach, although both the executive and working groups and the community members seemed content to be guided by the researchers on technical issues. This leads to the third point, that lack of experience of evaluation on the part of the community members and project staff and lack of experience of community development by the part-time researcher made each group slightly uncertain of the value of the various potential approaches to evaluation. Thus the aim was to produce a new, collaborative approach to evaluation between those involved in the day-to-day aspects of the project and those with experience in research. It was not to be the traditional evaluation of a project by outside academics.

The evaluation was planned to achieve some results over a short time-scale but also to provide information which could be used as the basis for a longer-term evaluation. The topics for evaluation were initially suggested by the researchers and subsequently agreed by the working group.

The community health volunteer project was identified as an important area of evaluation because it was a novel idea and one likely to be of interest to other community groups. It was also decided to monitor the use and usefulness of the Health Resource Library because it was an area of direct contact with the community and one in which the community health volunteers were likely to be directly involved. Furthermore, this evaluation would be straightforward and was likely to yield results which could be of direct use to the project staff. Finally, collaboration with other professional groups was considered by both the researchers and the working group to be a fundamental aspect of the project although one which would be more difficult to evaluate.

One aspect, suggested by the working group but not immediately taken on by the researchers, was evaluation of the effectiveness of the project's publicity. While the researchers accepted that this was an important and relevant area to monitor because of the dependence of the project on people getting to know about it, the resources available did not allow it to be included. However, the working group and the volunteers considered it so important that it subsequently formed the basis of a door-to-door survey by the volunteers.

Also discussed was the assessment of input to the project by the working group members, their perceptions of their own achievements and obstacles to their participation which were encountered in practice. While the working group agreed with the researcher on the importance of this aspect of the project, they were concerned that they had insufficient time to complete regular diaries throughout the first year. The eventual compromise was that a retrospective analysis of the minutes of working group meetings would replace this part of the evaluation.

All of the methods to be used were proposed by the researchers and agreed by the working group who were kept informed of progress at their regular meetings. Some methods were tailored in light of previous experiences of the project staff. For example, the use of a visitors' book to record all visits to the library was supplemented by a form on which details of visits were recorded by volunteers and project staff because it was felt that the visitors' book would not be comprehensive. However, this facilitated the recording of further information such as purpose and outcome of the visit and demographic information. The researcher collaborated with the project staff in the design of the data collection forms and suggested the acquisition of a computerized database for storage and analysis of the data. The computer subsequently proved to be popular with the volunteers. At a later stage, the researcher analysed the raw data with the project staff, showing them how to summarize the data in a way which would be of use in their own internal evaluations. When the data on use of the library was analysed at the end of year one, further publicity was prepared for those groups which were shown to be under-using the resource.

Community health volunteers were recruited and offered a training course. The subsequent role of the volunteers had not been fully determined, partly because their deployment depended to a great extent on their individual talents and interests.

The progress of this part of the project was monitored by semi-structured interviews when the volunteers were recruited and at intervals afterwards. The aim was to describe the volunteers' perceptions of their potential and actual role. The interviews included questions on the activities considered suitable, unsuitable and not liked, anticipated barriers to participation and the extent of collaboration with and support from other groups within and outside the project.

In the first year, each volunteer had two interviews. Both the interviews were semi-structured with specific questions as prompts. Every interviewee was asked the same specific questions although the order may have been slightly different to avoid breaking the flow of conversation if information was offered at an earlier stage in the interview. In both interviews, a completely open request for comments was made at the end. An attempt was made to encourage the volunteer to understand that their opinions would be used to improve the project as well as to chart its progress. Some of the information obtained from the interviews is presented later.

After discussion with the working group, it was decided to feed back the aggregated information from the interviews to the volunteers and to encourage discussion about perceived achievements, failures and obstacles in the project's first year in an informal discussion session. The opportunity was also taken to describe the purpose behind the evaluation and to invite questions. The executive and working groups, as well as the volunteers were invited to this meeting; however, none of the executive group were able to attend. The researcher's opinion was that the volunteers greatly appreciated this opportunity both to understand the evaluation and to discuss issues that were causing concern. The recorded achievements were greater than some volunteers had expected and several obstacles to full participation of volunteers in the project were identified and subsequently dealt with. Furthermore, several volunteers expressed satisfaction at knowing what the evaluation was seeking to achieve and how it was progressing as well as in being able to influence aspects of its planning. It was unanimously agreed that this type of meeting should be held more frequently. In the second year of the pilot, three-monthly evaluation meetings were planned.

To monitor the perceptions of other groups and to assess their views on the volunteer project, interviews of several professional groups (general practitioners, health visitors), the public and the executive and working groups were planned. Because of limited time, only the general practitioners were interviewed in year one. The perceptions of this group were considered important by the researchers, particularly because they had been identified by working group members as one of the most challenging groups to involve. However, the usefulness of obtaining these perceptions was not fully agreed on by the working group. The results indicated a high degree of interest from general practitioners but some scepticism as to the eventual effectiveness of the project.

It was originally intended that the general public would also be interviewed or surveyed in year one; however, the working group felt that this would be premature within the first twelve months of the project and, hence, this was delayed until year two.

Although assessing the effectiveness of publicity was not considered essential by the researchers, it was clearly important to members of the working group and to the volunteers who continued to raise the issue at the working group meetings. Therefore, it was suggested by the researcher that the volunteers design and carry out a survey of local residents. This was enthusiastically pursued by a few interested volunteers who formed a publicity subcommittee and enlisted the help of the researcher in designing data collection forms and in choosing a sample. The items of data to be collected were principally selected by the volunteers and the layout of the form, although initially prepared by the researcher due to lack of alternative resources, was piloted and altered in line with the volunteers' suggestions. For example, a statement was added at the beginning to remind each interviewer of a suitable form of introduction and an explanation of why the information was required. The volunteers prepared a rota system to cover several local streets and completed a door-to-door survey, aiming for approximately 100 households. The researcher analysed the data and presented the findings to the volunteers and project staff. Several positive effects were generated by this self-initiated study: the volunteers were very interested in the survey results and immediately began discussion of ways to improve their publicity, they expressed satisfaction at being able to carry through this piece of useful work and they appreciated the opportunity to talk to people about the project and to find out their opinions on its usefulness.

SOME RESULTS OF THE INITIAL EVALUATION

Many of these findings are particularly useful as baseline information against which to measure any change as the project proceeds. However, the descriptive information was also interesting and proved useful to the project staff and working group. Some of the information generated by the interviews of volunteers and by the publicity survey is now presented to give a flavour of the type of information obtained.

Although eighty-three people initially expressed interest in becoming volunteers, only twenty-six went through the training course and twenty were interviewed. The development of the volunteer role was slower than anticipated but by the end of the year, a framework for their training and deployment had been drawn up by the project staff and they had become involved in the development and the evaluation of the project. Even though the number of active volunteers decreased throughout the year, those who remained became involved in various activities including running self-help groups, attending conferences, developing the publicity strategy, writing a newsletter, compiling inserts for the local newspaper, providing information in the library and attending meetings of the executive group, the working group and local health forums.

Two groups of ten volunteers were interviewed: group A who were recruited in October and group B who were recruited the following February. Group A were interviewed when they had completed approximately half of their training course while seven of group B had attended one training session and the remaining three of group B had no training before the first interview. The second interview was carried out approximately six to nine months later; by this time, of the original twenty volunteers, four had left the area, one was working, one was on a placement and four had not been in touch with the project for several months. Therefore, nine volunteers (three males and six females) were available for the second interview and one more (female) was apparently still involved in the project. Five of those given a second interview were from the first ten volunteers recruited. The following is a summary of both interviews.

All twenty volunteers were from the local community; there were fifteen women and two were further education students. Eight people had volunteered after contact with the project for various reasons, including working on the local health profile which was carried out by community workers and local people participating in a Health Walk, attending a course offered by the project or contacting it for advice or to start a self-help group. Three people were already involved in voluntary work. Two people claimed that the project gave them something to do, three had health problems with which they had come to terms and wanted to help others do the same, two wanted to increase their own knowledge and one person hoped that working on the project would help in a future career.

Ten volunteers were already very involved with other local groups. These included self-help groups, other volunteer work, action/information groups and school/nursery groups. Six had been previously involved in other groups.

In total, five types of activity were initially suggested as suitable by the volunteers among a total of twenty-four individual activities. Five people suggested visiting people in their homes; ten suggested talking to people, individually or in groups, to give advice or suggest further contacts; three were particularly interested in setting up self-help groups; three were interested in giving out information leaflets and three in helping others, for example, by doing housework, shopping for the elderly and taking children or disabled people swimming.

The original twenty volunteers identified five types of activities as unsuitable. There was most agreement on counselling or dealing with people individually which was mentioned twice in each group. Group A identified more unsuitable activities than group B possibly because they had more time to think about the issues. Twenty activities were classed as personal dislikes. Thirteen volunteers mentioned groups with whom they lacked confidence or interest in dealing; these were people with depression, drug users, women, elderly people, disabled people, people with HIV or with alcohol problems (those unwilling to deal with women's problems were male).

The activities actually engaged in between the interviews by the nine volunteers were the publicity survey, talking to people at an occasional stall set up in a local market and in the library, attending meetings, helping self-help groups and organizing the library and office. Activities in which they had originally expressed an interest but which they had been unable to do were home visiting, talking to schools and associations, taking children and old people out and some self-help groups. These were all mentioned as activities they would like to do. Activities they liked, which were not mentioned at the first interview but arose during involvement in the project, were working with the computer, assisting with the planning of the new health centre, taking up the issue of dampness and involvement in the management of the project.

It is interesting to note that, despite the project orientation which has a strong emphasis on health promotion, this was not identified as a suitable or desirable task by volunteers; there was much more concern over coping with problems. This might indicate that volunteers started out with a relatively narrow definition of health; the project staff felt that this narrow definition broadened with continued involvement in the project.

Seven problems were anticipated at the outset as likely to cause difficulty in carrying out volunteer activities; the most common was lack of time which concerned nine of the twenty volunteers. The others related to lack of confidence, lack of status and lack of knowledge. Problems which did, in practice, hinder volunteer work were identified as mainly due to organizational problems and difficulties in getting projects off the ground, lack of an identified space for volunteers to relax and work in, lack of transport and lack of a crèche. Interestingly, none of the previously identified problems were realized by the nine who remained as volunteers.

When, at the second interview, the volunteers were asked to state the aim of the project, the replies were that it was to make people more aware, more empowered and to improve their health. Four of the nine volunteers felt that the project was achieving this aim but one volunteer thought the achievement was only with certain community groups. The other five volunteers complained of slowness, bureaucracy within the project and poor publicity compromising the achievements. Further spontaneous comments included disappointment that the project had been unable to help a member of the public with their problem as much as the volunteer had expected it to and that visitors to the library were too few. However, involvement in the project had given volunteers confidence and status in the community, for example, they were now invited to local meetings.

Volunteers were asked their perceptions about collaboration with three groups: other volunteers, working group members and the project executive group members. All said they had good links with the regular volunteers, although one suggested they saw one another a bit too often. Two felt they had good relationships with most of the working group, partly because of previous associations; three felt they had reasonable links with a few of the working group members while the remaining four felt they did not know this group at all. None of the volunteers felt they knew the project executive group at all.

Collaborations between volunteers and outside groups were wide-ranging, including links with other community groups and with health visitors.

For example, nine new links had been formed between volunteers and local groups such as the women's health group, the HIV workers' group and an alcoholics' group.

At the second interview, five volunteers felt that they were less positive about the project than they had been at the start while three were more positive and one was just the same. The reasons given for disillusionment were that the project's aim seemed to have been lost, that the project was moving too slowly and that there was little for volunteers to do. Reasons why individuals felt more positive were that they understood the project's aims better and felt more a part of the project. The volunteers' frustration was acknowledged by the project staff who had emphasized publicity, recruitment and training in year one; the framework for deployment of volunteers became a priority in year two.

At the start, fifteen volunteers rated themselves to be in fairly good to excellent health, three considered their health not very good and two poor. At the second interview, reported perceptions of their own health had improved in almost every case. At the first interview one of the nine had reported very good health, two good, four fairly good and two poor; at the second interview, there were two in very good health, five good and two fairly good. Seven of the nine felt that, by the second interview, they had made changes in their own life because of their involvement with the project; four had changed to a healthier diet with less meat, less salt and fewer sweets for the children, one person had lost a lot of weight, one took more exercise, one went out more and also had a greater interest in other activities, two felt more assertive, confident and aware but had made no changes in lifestyle and the last person had noted no difference at all.

In the publicity survey, eighty-eight people were interviewed of whom sixty-seven were female. Only 20 per cent were under twenty-four or over sixty-five years old. Twenty-two people (25 per cent) had heard of the project and all but one of these was female. Where the source of information was known it was, in order of popularity: the local newspaper, the playgroup, the community centre, the general practitioner's surgery or a friend. Eight people had visited the library, mostly to borrow books, while eleven knew of someone else who had visited. Twelve had heard about the Women's Health Week but only four had attended.

The only source of information to which regular exposure appeared to result in greater awareness of the project was the local clinic with 35 per cent of the regular female attenders being aware of the Women's Health Week compared with around 25 per cent of regular library attenders and regular newspaper readers. Overall, 53 per cent felt that they could use the project. Women were more likely to feel that they could use it (58 per cent) compared with men (38 per cent). The reasons given by people as to why they might not be able to use the project were varied and included both being too ill and being too healthy!

The volunteers were disappointed that so few of those surveyed had heard of the project; however, they had encountered a lot of interest during the survey. They felt that this experience had increased their enthusiasm for visiting local people in their own homes, for example, to give out information and to publicize the project. They also collected information on the newspapers which people read regularly and the services they visited which they intended to use to improve the project's publicity strategy.

CONCLUSIONS

This was an interesting and useful experience for all those involved. The project working group, the volunteers and the researchers felt that this project had broken some new ground for them in evolving a partnership between researchers and subjects and in making the evaluation fully a part of the project. The working group could see the relevance of the research as the evaluation proceeded, particularly at the end of the first year when they could use the results to improve the project and could build on the participative evaluation meetings which had been set up.

In deciding, initially, on the areas to be evaluated, it was clear that the working group and the researchers differed in their perceptions of the purpose and potential of the evaluation. The eventual evaluation was, to some extent, a compromise between each group's identified priorities and the resources available in terms of researcher's time. Further, at a later stage, the volunteers also became sufficiently confident to voice their own opinions on this aspect of the project. It is very likely that in a project of this nature, there will be several, perhaps equally valid, purposes for the evaluation and, hence, discussion, participation and collaboration between all relevant groups may need to be built in from the start with time allowed for the familiarization of those who are new to these ideas.

Furthermore, the volunteers in particular had difficulty in accepting the limitations of existing research methods in answering questions such as whether the project would have a significant effect on the health of the local community. While they could see the worth of process measures which assisted them in improving the day-to-day operation of the project, they also wanted to be able to measure improvements in health outcomes or such variables as the number of people in the community eating healthier diets compared with previously.

Several positive effects of the evaluation which had not been anticipated were noted. These were that

1 as the evaluation proceeded, it involved, to some extent, most of those in the working group, the project staff and the volunteers; this allowed everyone to identify with and use the results
2 when the findings from the interviews with volunteers were summarized and presented, the resulting discussion sessions allowed problems to be aired and, often, resolved
3 the evaluation itself developed during the first year as ideas were generated and the second-year pilot study was to include areas not previously tackled
4 evaluation became an integral part of the project and, to some extent, a driving force; it may even have become a mechanism for achieving some of the project aims, for example, empowerment of the volunteers
5 finally, funding was obtained to allow an experienced health promotion officer to undertake a further research study, developing evaluation methods which can be used in this type of project.

Chapter 12

Healthy Cities

A modern problem or a post-modern solution?

Michael P. Kelly, John K. Davies and Bruce G. Charlton

In this chapter we argue that if the Healthy Cities movement retains a commitment to conventional, discipline-bound research methods and paradigms, it will not only remain irrelevant to the mainstream delivery of acute and chronic medical services, but also, and more importantly, it will not succeed even in its own intersectoral and participative mission. Some of the contributors to this volume have demonstrated how research for Healthy Cities, the new public health or community development may become marginalized. Other contributors have shown just how difficult it can be, even when research concerned with Healthy Cities is not sidelined. We suggest that the reasons for this lie not in a conspiracy to disparage this type of research. Rather, we argue that the concept of Healthy Cities and its underlying philosophical principle of Health for All are simply incompatible with conventional discipline-led models of scientific research and rational administration. We also suggest that the implications of that incompatibility must be grasped for the vision of Healthy Cities to be realized.

Conventional scientific research and the Healthy Cities concept belong to two fundamentally different worlds: the modern and the post-modern. Modernity is the world of conventional scientific research and rational administration applied to problems, physical or social. Post-modernity is a world of aesthetics, of the deconstruction of conventional social arrangements, and of experimentation in cultural, artistic and life forms (Lyotard 1984; Bauman 1992; Featherstone 1988). The Healthy Cities movement is one such experiment. The core idea of post-modernity is that the social and moral conditions pertaining in the world at the present time mark a fundamental break with the past. In art, form displaces content; in philosophy, interpretation displaces system; in politics, pragmatism displaces principle; and in science chaos displaces order. To be paradoxical: the core idea of post-modernity is that there are no core ideas! In Healthy Cities, an emphasis on health displaces an emphasis on disease, in research for Healthy Cities the focus should be on the origins of health rather than the origins of disease.

Albeit unwittingly, the depiction of health established in the WHO 1946 definition (WHO 1946) – a state of complete physical, mental and social well-being, and not merely the absence of disease or infirmity – created the original post-modern motif for health. We say 'unwittingly' because WHO in its practice and its personnel has generally been an ultra-modernist organization, favouring technical expertise as a means of solving clearly defined problems. It is true that advocates of the health promotion movement frequently describe their activities as constituting a decisive break with the medically dominated model of health (De Leeuw 1989b), yet they may have identified the wrong decisive break! Conventionally, the social model of health is contrasted with the traditional medical model in this context. We contend, following Antonovsky (1984; 1985; 1987), that both the social *and* medical models remain locked in a pathogenic (and modernist) world-view. Pathogenesis seeks out the underlying causes of *system breakdown*. Both the social and medical models are united by a commitment to the existence of a system which is capable of being destroyed, broken down and analysed. The fact that one model identifies microbiological pathogens, and the other social pathogens, is not a fundamental difference (Antonovsky 1987; Kelly 1989; 1990a). Both models are based upon a causal epistemology whereby bad outcomes have bad precursors and the job of the scientist – social or medical – is to identify the ways of eliminating, or controlling, the pathogen.

The post-modern approach does not see or seek systems. It views physical and social life as chaotic and their understanding as contingent. Antonovsky's position challenges us to address not the origins of pathology, but the origins of health. This Antonovsky calls salutogenesis. Salutogenesis is critical for Healthy Cities for two reasons. First, it defines the goal or purpose as understanding the origins of health. Second, its focus upon survival in spite of inbuilt tendencies to chaos, disorder and fragmentation is capable of uniting disciplines as diverse as Sociology and Anatomy and Anthropology and Epidemiology. Science in the post-modern condition is concerned with discipline integration not discipline imperialism.

Our premise, then, is that it is not the social model of health which is the basis of the difference between conventional approaches and the new public health and the Healthy Cities movement. The social and medical models are both system-based, and built upon the assumption that an underlying system is open to systematic scientific explanation and investigation. We suggest that the distinction between this and the philosophy of

Healthy Cities, Health for All and health promotion more generally, is the emphasis on *positive health*. Positive health is the key and post-modern concept in this regard. But positive health is not amenable to conventional scientific investigation, or to conventional (modern) scientific discussion (Charlton and Kelly 1992b).

The paradigm which stalks much work on Healthy Cities, health promotion and the new public health is that of 'normal' science. Normal science is convergent and has a defined object, methodology and procedure for validation (Kuhn 1970). It is hardly surprising that normal science is so seductive to Healthy Cities, given that normal science has such a long and distinguished track record. For many purposes, including most medical ones, it is the best available (Charlton, in press). Normal science is based on the assumption that if enough time, energy and resources are expended on a problem, then, inevitably, a scientific solution will be forthcoming. Normal science is a puzzle-solving exercise which works within a strong and accepted paradigm where we know what the problem is, and that there is an answer to it. The scientist's task is working out that answer.

This book has recorded a variety of attempts, some of which are normal science and some of which try to break out of normal science practice. All record the tensions, the difficulties and the problems of bringing together communities, researchers, policy-makers, and planners. But the difficulties recorded in this book stem from the fact that Healthy Cities work is not like a puzzle. Once communities are brought into the research process in a meaningful way, and scientists and other stakeholders no longer define conventional research problems, the nature of what the question should be and whose version of truth should be applied to evaluate the answer immediately become matters of dispute. The normal science paradigm is shattered. It is not clear what the answer might look like, whether we would know it if we found it or even whether the answer exists at all! This is not puzzle solving, it is not even a paradigm shift. It is turning the scientific enterprise upside down.

MODERNITY, POST-MODERNITY AND HEALTH

Post-modernity as a sociological, philosophical, cultural and artistic idea has many meanings (Giddens 1992). However, for the present purposes, it refers to a major social and cultural disjunction that has happened in various fields of human cultural and scientific endeavour particularly in the twentieth century. This has been associated with the discrediting and questioning of the possibility of ultimate truth and/or human happiness being revealed or produced by science. Cities which are largely the result of human planning with their urban sprawls, their pollution, their social problems and their inequalities in health seem to give the lie to the fact that rationalist planning can produce human happiness.

Modernity defines itself in contrast to the traditional order, and implies a progressive economic and administrative rationalization and differentiation of the social world. Post-modernity suggests an epochal shift or break with this, involving the growth of a new social totality with distinct emerging principles (Featherstone 1988). Instead of progress we have just change – the ultimate goal or telos is lost. In a cultural sense, post-modernity emphasizes aesthetic self-consciousness, a rejection of system in favour of simultaneity, montage and pastiche, and the paradoxical, ambiguous and uncertain open-ended nature of reality (Featherstone 1988).

Modernity was based on a fundamental belief that there was an absolute bedrock of rational truth upon which scientific and rational inquiry was converging (Kellner 1988 : 240). From Elizabethan times onwards in Britain, for example, the guiding assumption in the provision of services related to health and welfare was precisely this: that there is a truth discernible through scientific or other rational endeavour. That there have actually been many different rationalities is not taken, and historically has not been taken, to mean that the search for an ultimate solution was wrong, merely that one's political or scientific opponents were misguided, deluded, immoral, dishonest or plain wrong.

The post-modern view, which is implicit in the principle of Health for All, is relativist. It does not seek ultimate truths about health, it simply acknowledges that positive health is a quality of individuals and social groups that is self-defined, not externally imposed. The original WHO definition of health is often derided. In rationalist terms, quite rightly so – it is meaningless. What, for example, is complete social well-being? How would we measure it? Of course, it is unmeasurable! It is subjective and belongs to, and is the property of, the individual or group and is not the possession of some scientist or administrator who wants to control or operationalize it. Once this is grasped, the fact that it cannot be measured in the same way that pathology can be measured ceases to be a problem.

Dubos (1962) heralded similar ideas when he described health as a pattern of adjustment or adaptation within the environment. 'Health is the expression of the extent to which the individual and social body maintain in readiness the resources required to meet the exigencies of the future,' (Dubos 1962). According to Nutbeam (1986), within the context of health promotion, health has been considered less as an abstract state and more in terms of the ability to achieve potential and to respond positively to the challenges of one's environment. In these terms, health is seen as a resource for everyday life, not merely the objective of living. It is a positive concept emphasizing social and personal, as well as physical, capacities. Such a view emphasizes the interaction between individuals and their environment and the need to achieve some balance between the two (De Leeuw 1989b). The post-modern vision of health is founded, therefore, in aesthetics and in moral values. In the post-modern condition, aesthetic considerations are, whether we like it or not, paramount in determining how we choose to lead or shape our own lives and how we assess what is a good life (Shustermann 1988: 355). If we are to develop a post-modern healthy city in which we can practise Health for All and in which the new public health can thrive, the importance of this definition must be recognized, although the whole notion of producing a healthy city by rational planning is precisely, of course, what is at issue!

The definitions of Dubos and Nutbeam amount to a rejection of the notion of health as the opposite of disease. Health and disease are not to be conceptualized as two ends of a continuous spectrum. Disease and health belong to quite separate universes of discourse, one modern, the other post-modern. Healthy Cities will, therefore, sit most uneasily within that most modern of scientific discourses, namely scientific medicine. Historically speaking, the definitions of positive health gained popularity precisely at the point when the critique of rationalist medicine reached a crescendo in the 1960s and 1970s. Writers as diverse as Illich (1975) Szaz (1972), McKeown (1976) and others in their different ways questioned the underlying rationalist and normative principles of medical advance. Sociologists in particular highlighted the role of medicine as an instrument of social control (Friedson 1970). The arguments about medical dominance, medical imperialism, the limitations of high technology medicine and so on, were vigorously debated a generation or so ago. Much of the debate eventually metamorphosed into doctor-bashing. In practice, much of this doctor-bashing was probably misguided, not because doctors did not deserve criticism, but because it missed the main point (Kelly 1990b). What the Healthy Cities vision offers is a way out of the now sterile debates of the 1960s and a genuinely integrated approach to health promotion. The role of research in such an endeavour hinges not on its methodology and whether such methodology is qualitative or quantitative. The role of research depends first, on its ability to embrace its objects of study (i.e., ordinary people) in its own processes; second, its capacity to work across traditional and conventional discipline boundaries; and third, its willingness to recognize the chaotic, contingent and non-systemic nature of social and physical reality.

The point of departure for the unification of research and practice in

Healthy Cities is an emphasis on health as a phenomenon which is subjectively defined and must include biological, social, psychological and environmental factors. What the Healthy Cities movement must articulate rapidly, is a means of integrating these levels of analysis in a way which the modernist boundaries between sociology, medicine, psychology and the environmental sciences are dissolved. This dissolution is entirely in line with the spirit of the post-modern condition in which the very subject matter is contingent. Here the existence of a systemic universe governed by underlying laws amenable to scientific investigation is rejected in favour of a view of knowledge which must constantly modify itself, must be tentative, probalistic and reversible (Kellner 1988). Such knowledge changes and develops but does not have a transcendental goal.

Modernity was the attempt to impose structures on a disorderly world (Bauman 1992). Post-modernity is the celebration of disorderliness and the recognition of the impossibility of anything other than imperfect and temporary structures of meaning being imposed upon the disordered world. The history of the delivery of health services and the organization of towns and cities has been precisely the searching after human systems of perfection in the face of individual people with their own minds, and patterns of social and medical problems which defy easy solution of any kind. The Healthy Cities project and the Health for All movement must acknowledge that systems of perfection (including their own) are modern utopian inventions, and that human happiness is not so much a product of human institutions, but more a product of human relationships. In pessimistic mood Bauman argues that post-modern society is one in which the place previously dominated by human work is now dominated by consumer life (Bauman 1992: 51). Pleasure is no longer a diversion from reality, pleasure *is* reality, and freedom is the choice between greater and lesser satisfactions in the market place. Fashion has a pervasive role in post-modern society and the market is based upon meeting the needs of rapidly changing fashion. If society is based upon desire – including the desire for physical, psychological and social well-being – then desire must be refreshed and sharpened by novelty. The fads for healthy foods, diets, aerobics are also part of the search for novelty. In these circumstances, health is not so much an economic good, but is a private choice (Charlton and Kelly 1992a). It is not something which is imposed upon individuals by some national or local organization (the traditional public health model), but something which people choose for themselves from a range of goods on offer – 'making healthy choices the easy choices' in the jargon of healthy public policy, or the bottom–up approach.

Jean-François Lyotard, the super pundit of post-modernity, has argued that post-modernity is about an attack on the two great Western scientific and philosophical traditions which developed out of the Enlightenment: that of the liberation of humanity and that of the speculative unity of knowledge. The post-modern condition is a state of mind, or an attitude, which calls into question these grand myths or 'metanarratives' (Lyotard 1984). Of course the Healthy Cities movement, the research reported in this book and the Health for All principles, share to a large extent these great Enlightenment concerns. They are driven both by a desire for greater equality, or at least an attempt to combat inequalities in health, and by the notion that scientific or rational principles could lead society in that direction. But, if it is to be successful, they must be something both more and less than that.

Lyotard identified the relationship between science and politics as crucial in the period of modernity. In the modern world, he argued, science and reason legitimated power relations. In the post-modern condition, science and reason no longer legitimate politics and power. Scientific discussion becomes marginalized, as it fragments into a range of disciplines and sub-disciplines between which meaningful communications become impossible. The political process, meanwhile, finds its legitimation in a consumer led market economy of constantly evolving images, media and novelty. The tendency for the disciplines and sub-disciplines which can make a contribution to understanding the origins of health, like medical sociology, health psychology, microbiology, biochemistry, environmental health, infection control, epidemiology, and so on, to fragment into an increasing number of isolated factions jostling for supremacy and each claiming its own particular version of social or physical reality as the most appropriate, is but one example of the post-modern condition. The apparent marginality of much, if not all, of the activities of such experts to mainstream policy-making about the health service in Britain in the 1990s for example, seems to bear out Lyotard's thesis.

Healthy Cities and Health for All are political as well as scientific activities. The principles of the Ottawa Charter (WHO 1986) are political principles, not conventional scientific ones; demands for the prerequisites of health are political not scientific, and the doctrine of positive health is an aesthetic and moral principle not a scientific one! In such political processes meta-narratives (to use Lyotard's terms) must give way to 'micro-narratives'. More precisely the post-modern science for Health for All and Healthy Cities must attempt to describe the lives of men and women as they live and experience them (Kelly 1990a; 1990c; 1992). It must grasp the complexities of their thoughts and actions as they move through stressor-rich environments and attempt to come to some kind of accommodation with them. That accommodation with them will be microbiological and internal. It will be macro-biological *vis-à-vis* the external world. It will be psychological and interpersonal. It will be a political, economic and geological process more akin to the flexible, goal-directed micro-analysis of advertising and marketing than to the abstract, principled analysis of science. For the purposes of understanding these adaptation processes, it is useless to abstract. Abstraction is a modernist principle. The post-modern solution integrates the holistic involvement in all these spheres of human existence and states that they must be understood in themselves and in the way the individual understands them him or herself. Only then may micro-narrative goals be successfully achieved.

Healthy Cities could be viewed as merely yet another separate rationality which, while distinctive, follows a pattern discernible from the time of the Enlightenment. Its attack on inequalities and its scientific credo strongly suggest that many of its advocates see it in precisely these terms, as a superior rationalist solution to a set of hitherto insuperable problems. If that were, or is, the case, when the history of the delivery of health care comes to be written a hundred years from now, Healthy Cities will merit at best a footnote among the avalanche of late twentieth century attempts to get things right. However, if the truly post-modern conception of Healthy Cities is grasped with its emphasis on the values of locality and community, aestheticism, relativism and private behaviour, then it will mark a turning point in the history of our understanding of health.

These kinds of ideas are not new. The philosophy of Schutz (1967), the ecology of Dubos (1980), the sociology of Antonovsky (1985) and the psychology of Lazarus (1980) all in their ways, contribute to this view. The fundamental break with conventional science that each of these writers make, and the implications of their work for Healthy Cities, has not made much progress yet. But there is hope. Much of what has been described in this book has consisted of attempts to develop ways round the difficulties of applying research to practice. Antonovsky's work has been given some prominence in the volume and his concept of salutogenesis – the study of the origins of health – was indeed a seminal principle which the early writers on Healthy Cities made reference to. We would like to see Antonovsky's work receive still more prominence. We would like, too, to see models and theories of change – for Healthy Cities is a movement about change – which have an integrated approach to the potential contributing disciplines, being developed. We would like to see many more experiments of involvement and participation, not in narrowly partisan ways, but in ways that allow the wit and wisdom of ordinary men and women to sit comfortably with the knowledge accumulated by conventional scientific methods.

Of course, post-modernity is only one part of the picture. Boundaries and limitations will remain in science, in medicine and even in artistic and political discourse (Charlton, in press). But the post-modern mood is powerful and pervasive. If the Healthy Cities movement is able to come to terms with the post-modern condition – both in exploring its rich inner possibilities, and in becoming aware of its inherent contradictions – this can only strengthen its available strategies for future development. A consideration of post-modernity can teach us not so much the right answers, but how *not* to ask the wrong questions.

References

Ackernecht E. (1981) *Rudolf Virchow*, Arno Press, New York.

Adams, L., Smithies, J., with Beattie, A., Webster, G. (1990) *Community Participation and Health Promotion*, HEA, London.

Anderson, R., Davies, J. K., Kickbusch, I., McQueen, D. V. and Turner, J. (eds) (1988) *Health Behaviour Research and Health Promotion*, Oxford University Press, Oxford.

Antonovsky, A. (1984) 'The sense of coherence as a determinant of health', *Advances* 1: 37–50.

—— (1985) *Health, Stress and Coping*, Jossey Bass, San Francisco.

—— (1987) *Unravelling the Mystery of Health: How People Manage Stress and Stay Well*, Jossey Bass, San Francisco.

Anyanwu, C. N. (1988) 'The techniques of participatory research', *Community Development Journal* 23: 11–15.

APEX/PH (1991) *Assessment Protocol for Excellence in Public Health: A Workbook*, National Association of County Health Officials, Washington, D C.

Ashton, J. (ed.) (1992) *Healthy Cities*, Open University Press, Milton Keynes.

Baum, F. (1986) 'Assessing community health needs: pitfalls, practicalities and a proposed model'. Paper presented at the Second Australian Family Research Conference, Melbourne, 26th–28th November.

—— (1988) 'Community based research for promoting the new public health', *Health Promotion International* 3: 259–68.

—— (1990) 'The new public health: force for change or reaction?', *Health Promotion International* 5: 145–50.

Baum, F. and Abbott, D. (1989) *Social Health Report: Marion, Brighton and Glenelg Community Health Needs Assessment*, Southern Community Health Research Unit, Adelaide.

Baum, F. and Brown, V. (1989) 'Healthy Cities (Australia) project: issues of evaluation for the new public health', *Community Health Studies* 13: 140–9.

Baum, F. and Cooke, R. (1992) 'Healthy Cities Australia: the evaluation of the pilot project in Noarlunga, South Australia', *Health Promotion International* 7: 181–93.

Baum, F., Cooke, R., Crowe, K., Traynor, M., Clarke, B. (1990) *Evaluation of the Healthy Cities Noarlunga Project*, Southern Community Health Research Unit, South Australia Health Commission, Adelaide.

Bauman, Z. (1992) *Intimations of Postmodernity*, Routledge, London.

Bayless, H. (1983) *The Best Towns in America*, Houghton Mifflin, Boston.

Beattie, A. (1991) 'Knowledge and control in health promotion: a test case for social theory', in J. Gabe, M. Calnan and M. Bury, (eds) *The Sociology of the Health Service*, Routledge, London.

Bell, C. and Newby, H. (1971) *Community Studies*, George Allen & Unwin, London.

Benz, L. N. (1975) 'Citizen participation, reconsidered', *Social Work* March: 115–19.

Bethell, C. (1991) 'Is the community health profile necessary?', *Health Visitor* 64: 294–6.

Bowling, A. (1991) *Measuring Health*, Open University Press, Milton Keynes.

Bracht, N. (ed.) (1990) *Health Promotion at the Community Level*, Sage, Beverly Hills.

Briggs, A. (1968) *Victorian Cities*, Penguin, London.

Brinberg, D. and McGrath, J. E. (1985) *Validity and the Research Process*, Sage, Beverly Hills.

Brooke, J. (1990) 'But the point is to change the world!' (Paper delivered at a conference on Housing and Health: Time for Action), Royal Institute of Public Health and Hygiene, St. Bartholomew's Hospital, London.

Bulmer, M. (1986) *Social Science & Social Policy*, Allen & Unwin, London.

Byrne, D. (1991) 'Divided cities – unhealthy cities', (paper presented at the British Sociological Association Annual Conference, Manchester, March).

Cabinet Office (1990) *Annual review of government-funded research and development*, HMSO, London.

California Healthy Cities Project, (1990) California Healthy Cities Project, Sacramento, CA.

Canadian Journal of Public Health (1985): 'Beyond Health Care', *Canadian Journal of Public Health* Supplement 1.

Cappon, D. (1990) 'Indicators for a Healthy City', *Environmental Management and Health* 1: 9–18.

Cardinal, L. et O'Neill, M. (1992) 'Une bibliographie annotée sur des indicateurs pour évaluer les projets de Villes et villages en santé', in M. O'Neill and L. Cardinal (eds) (1992) *Des indicateurs pour évaluer les projets québécois de Villes et villages en santé; la nécessité de faire des choix*; Quebéc, Groupe de recherche et d'intervention en promotion de la santé de l'Université Laval (GRIPSUL), DSC de l'Hôpital de l'Enfant Jésus et DSC de l'Hôpital St-Sacrement: 128–34.

Cawson, A. (1982) *Corporatism & Welfare, Social Policy and State Invervention in Britain*, Heinemann, London.

Centres for Disease Control (1991) *A Guide to the Selection and Utilization of Selected Health Assessment and Planning Models to Improve Community Health and Contribute to the Achievement of the Year 2000 Objectives* US Department of Health and Human Services, Public Health Service, Centres for Disease Control Atlanta, Georgia.

Charlton, B. G. (in press) 'Medicine and post-modernity', *Journal of the Royal Society of Medicine*.

Charlton, B. G. and Kelly, M. P. (1992a) 'Profit and loss on the pulse of a nation', *The Times Higher Education Supplement*, 7 February 1992, 1005: 19.

Charlton, B. G. and Kelly, M. P. (1992b) 'Paying for an off-the-peg life', *The Times Higher Education Supplement*, 22 May 1992, 1020: 19.

Cohen, S. and Syne, S. (1985) (eds) *Social Support and Health*, Academic Press, Orlando.

Community Development and Health Project (1990) *Strengthening Community Health: Report of the Consultancy and Evaluation Project*, Victoria, Australia.

Cooke, R. and Skewes, A. (1990) 'Community perception and responses to environmental health issues in Noarlunga', (paper presented at the Third Australian Community Health Association Conference, Sydney, October).

Craig, N., Pederson, A., Rootman, I., Stirling, A. (1991) *Information for Planning Healthy Communities*, (proceedings of an invitational workshop), Ontario Prevention Clearinghouse, Toronto.

Crosswaite, C. and Curtice, L. (1991) 'Dissemination of research for health promotion, a literature review', Research Unit in Health and Behavioural Change, University of Edinburgh, Edinburgh.

Curtice, L. (1991) 'European Healthy Cities research – where is it?', *Critical Public Health*, 1: 42–8.

Curtice, L. and McQueen, D. V. (1990) *The WHO Healthy Cities Project – An Analysis of Progress*, Working Paper No. 40, Research Unit in Health and Behavioural Change, University of Edinburgh, Edinburgh.

Daghlian, S., Kelly, M. P., Dyce, G., O'Neill, M. (1992) *Unemployment and Health: A Case Study of Research, Community Development and Community Decline*, Glasgow: Community Health Resource Unit.

De Leeuw, E. (1989a) *Health Policy: An exploratory inquiry into the development of policy for the new public health in the Netherlands*, Savannah/Datawyse, Maastricht.

—— (1989b) *The Sane Revolution : Health Promotion :background scope, prospects*, Van Gorcum, Assen.

—— (1990) *Research for Healthy Cities Newsletter*, 1.

—— (ed.) (1991a) *Research for Healthy Cities Newsletter*, 2

De Leeuw, E., Breemer ter Stege, B., de Jong, G. A. (eds) (1990) *Proceedings of Research for Healthy Cities International Conference, the Netherlands*, Supplement TSG 11/90, Leiden: Vereniging voor Volksgezondheid en Wetenschap.

De Swaan, A. (1988) *In Care of the State*, Polity Press, Cambridge.

DeMarco, J. (1990) 'Knowledge for what?', (a paper presented at the First National Conference on Health Promotion Research, Toronto, November 1990), Centre for Health Promotion, University of Toronto.

Dekker, E. and Saan, H. (1990) 'Policy papers, papers or policies: HFA under uncertain political conditions', *Health Promotion International* 5: 279–90.

Delamothe, T. (1989) 'Statistics today: urgent need to depoliticize official figures', *British Medical Journal* 299: 1543–4.

Delaney, F. and Moran G. (1991) 'Collaboration for health: in theory and practice', *Health Education Journal* 50: 2, 97–9.

Department of Health and Social Security (1980) *Inequalities in health: report of a research working group*, DHSS, London.

Dickens, P. (1990) *Urban Sociology, Society, Locality and Human Nature*, Harvester Wheatsheaf, London.

Dixon, J. (1989) 'The limits and potential of community development for personal and social change', *Community Health Studies* 13: 82–92.

Dluhy, M. J. (1990) *Building Conditions in the Human Services*, London: Sage.

DoH/NHS Management Executive (1990), *Consultation and Involving the Consumer*, London.

Downie, R. S., Fyfe, C. and Tannahill, A. (1990) *Health Promotion Models and Values*, Oxford University Press, Oxford.

Dubos, R. (1962) *Torch of Life*, Simon and Schuster, New York.

—— (1980) *Man Adapting*, Yale University Press, New Haven.

Duhl, L. (1988) 'The Mind of the City – the Context of Urban Life', *Environments* 19: 1–13.

Dwyer, J. (1989) 'The politics of participation', *Community Health Studies* 13: 59–73.

Dye, T. R. (1972) *Understanding Public Policy*, Prentice Hall, Englewood Cliffs, New Jersey.

Epp, J. (1986a) *Stratégies nationales en promotion de la santé*; paper presented at the 77th conference of the Canadian Public Health Association, Vancouver, June.

—— (1986b) 'Achieving Health for All: a Framework for health promotion', *Health Promotion an International Journal* 1: 419–28.

Evers, A., Farrant, W. and Trojan, A. (1990) *Healthy Public Policy at the Local Level*, Campus/Westview, Frankfurt/Boulder.

Farrant, W. and Russell, J. (1986) *The Politics of Health Education* Bedford Way Paper 28, Institute of Education, University of London.

Feather, J. (1990) 'Prairie region workshop on indicators for healthy communities: a view in retrospect', unpublished paper presented at the First National Conference on Health Promotion Research, Toronto.

Feather, J. and Mathur, B. (eds) (1990) 'Indicators for Healthy Communities', proceedings of an invitational workshop; Saskatoon, Health Status Research Unit, Department of Community Health and Epidemiology, University of Saskatchewan.

Featherstone, M. (1988) 'In pursuit of the post-modern: an introduction', *Theory Culture and Society* 5: 195–215.

Feurstein, M.-T. (1986) *Partners in Evaluation: Evaluating Development and Community Programmes with Participants*, Macmillan, London.

—— (1988) 'Finding the methods to fit the people: training for participatory evaluation', *Community Development Journal* 23: 16–25.

Finch, J. (1986) *Research and Policy: The Uses of Qualitative Methods in Social and Educational Research*, Falmer, Brighton.

Flynn, B. C. (ed.) (1992) 'Healthy Cities in the United States', in Ashton, J. *Healthy Cities*, Open University Press, Milton Keynes.

Flynn, B. C., Rider, M. and Ray, D. W. (1991) 'Healthy Cities: the Indiana model of community development in public health', *Health Education Quarterly* 18: 331–47.

Flynn, B. C. and Rider, M. (1991) 'Healthy Cities Indiana: mainstreaming community health in the United States', *American Journal of Public Health* 81: 510–11.

Fortin, J. P., O'Neill, M., Lemieux, V., Groleau, G., Cardinal, L. and Racine, P. (1991) *Les conditions de réussite du mouvement québécois de Villes et villages en santé*; Réseau de recherche socio-politique et organisationnelle en santé de l'Université Laval et Unité de recherche en santé communautaire du Centre Hospitalier de l'Université Laval, Québec.

Friedson, E. (1970) *Professional Dominance: The Social Structure of Medical Care*, Aldine, Chicago.

Furler, E. (1979) 'Against hegemony in health care service evaluation', *Community Health Studies* 3: 32–41.

Gans, H. (1967) *The Levittowners*, Random House, New York.

Giddens, A. (1992) 'Uprooted signposts at the century's end', *The Times Higher Education Supplement* January 17: 21–2.

Glazer, N. (1988) *The Limits of Social Policy*, Harvard University Press, Cambridge, Massachusetts.

Green, L. W. and Kreuter, D. W. (1991) *Health Promotion Planning: an Educational and Environmental Approach*, Mayfield Publishers, Mountain View, California.

Guba, E. G. and Lincoln, Y. S. (1989) *Fourth Generation Evaluation*, Sage, Beverly Hills.

Gusfield, J. (1975) 'Categories of ownership and responsibility in social issues: alcohol abuse and automobile use', *Journal of Drug Issues* 5: 290–5.

Habermas, J. (1971) *Towards a Rational Society*, Heineman, London.

Hancock, T. (1985) 'The mandala of health: a model of the human ecosystem', *Family and Community Health* 8: 1–10.

Hancock, T. and Duhl, L. (1986) (WHO Healthy Cities Paper 1) *Healthy Cities: Promoting Health in the Urban Context*, FADL, Copenhagen.

Hayes, M. (1991) 'What kind of institute for what kind of health promotion?' *IHPR Bulletin*.

Hayes, M. and Manson-Willms, S. (1990) 'Healthy community indicators: the perils of the search and the paucity of the find', *Health Promotion* 5: 161–6.

Healey, P. (1990) 'Policy Processes in Planning', *Policy and Politics* 18: 91–103.

Health and Welfare Canada (HWC) (1989) *Knowledge Development for Health Promotion: a Call for Action*, Health and Welfare Canada, Health Services and Promotion Branch, Working paper 89–2, Ottawa.

Health and Welfare Canada (HWC) (1990) 'Developing Knowledge for Health Promotion in Canada', *Health Promotion/Promotion de la santé* 28 (special insert): 1–14.

Health Education Authority/Open University (1990) *Baseline Review of Community Development and Health Education*, Milton Keynes, Open University.

Health Promotion International (1989) 4, (contains several papers from the Healthy Cities Symposium in Zagreb).

Healthy Communities 2000: Model Standards (1991) American Public Health Association, Washington, DC.

Healthy People 2000, National Health Promotion and Disease Prevention Objectives (1990) Government Printing Office, Washington, DC.

Holman, B. (1987) 'Research from the underside', *British Journal of Social Work* 17: 669–83.

Hunt, S. (1987) 'Evaluating a community development project: issues of acceptability', *British Journal of Social Work* 17: 661–7.

—— (1990a) 'Emotional distress and bad housing', *Health and Hygiene* 11: 72–9.

—— (1990b) 'Building alliances: professional and political issues in community participation, Examples from a health and community development project', *Health Promotion International* 5: 179–85.

Hunt, S. and Lewis, L. (1989) 'Damp Housing, Mould Growth and Health Status, Part II. House mould and symptoms, Report to the funding bodies', University of Edinburgh.

Hunt, S., McEwen, J. and McKenna, S. D. (1986b) *Measuring Health Status*, Croom Helm, London.

Hunt, S., Martin, C. J. and Platt, S. (1986a) 'Report on a Study of Housing and Health Status', RUHBC, University of Edinburgh.

Hunt, S., Martin, C. J. and Platt, S. (1987) 'Housing and health in deprived areas of Edinburgh', in *Unhealthy Housing: A Diagnosis*. Proceedings of a conference. The Institute of Environmental Health Officers and the Legal Research Institute, University of Warwick.

Hunt, S. M., Martin, C. J., Platt, S. and Lewis, C. (1989) 'Damp Housing, Mould Growth and Health Status', Part I (report to the funding bodies), University of Edinburgh.

Ife, J. (1980) 'The determination of social need – a model of need statements in social administration', *Australian Journal of Social Issues* 15(2): 92–107.

Illich, I. (1975) *Medical Nemesis*, Calder and Boyars, London.

—— (1977) *Disabling Professions*, Marion Boyars, London.

Inner City Health Project (1990) *Final Evaluation Report*, Bristol.

Institute of Medicine (1988) *The Future of Public Health*, National Academy Press, Washington, DC.

Judd, D. and Parkinson, M. (eds) (1990) *Leadership and Urban Regeneration*, Sage, Beverly Hills.

Kalucy, L. (1989) *Older Person's Report: Marion, Brighton and Glenelg Community Health Needs Assessment*, Southern Community Health Research Unit, Adelaide.

Kaplan, R. (1988) 'The value dimension in studies of health promotion', in S. Spacapan and S. Oskamp (eds) *The Social Psychology of Health*, Sage, New York.

Kellner, D. (1988) 'Post-modernism as social theory: some challenges and problems', *Theory, Culture and Society* 5: 239–69.

Kelly, M. P. (1988) 'Workshop and Information Exchange on "Health for All"' *Social Research Association News* July/August 1988: 9–10.

—— (1989) 'Some problems in health promotion research', *Health Promotion* 4: 317–30.

—— (1990a) 'The role of research in the new public health', *Critical Public Health* 3: 4–9.

—— (1990b) 'A suitable case for technik: behavioural science in the post-graduate medical curriculum', *Medical Education* 24: 271–9.

—— (1990c) 'The World Health Organization's definition of health promotion: three problems', *Health Bulletin* 48: 176–80.

—— (1991) 'Research for "Health for All": the healthy city and its evaluation', *Research for Healthy Cities* 2 (newsletter of the Healthy Cities network, Quebec, Copenhagen, Edinburgh and Maastricht): 5–6.

—— (1992) Foreword, to A. Kennedy, *Local Voices Local Lives – the story of the Kendoon Community Health Profile*, Drumchapel Community Health Project, Glasgow.

Kickbusch, I. (1986) 'Health promotion, a global perspective', *Canadian Journal of Public Health* 77: 321–7.

—— (1987) 'Issues in health promotion', *Health Promotion* 1: 437–42.

—— (1989) 'Healthy Cities; a working project and a growing movement', *Health Promotion International* 4: 77–82.

Kuhn, T. (1970) *The Structure of Scientific Revolutions*, University of Chicago Press, second edition, Chicago.

Labonté, R. and Penfold, S. (1981) 'Analyse critique des perspectives canadiennes en promotion de la santé', *Education sanitaire* 19: 4–10.

Lalonde, M. (1974) *A New Perspective on the Health of Canadians*, Ministry of Supply and Services, Canadian Federal Government, Ottawa.

Lawler, E. E., Mohrman, A. M., Mohrman, S. A., Ledford, G. E., Cummings, T. G. and Associates (1985) *Doing Research that is Useful for Theory and Practice*, Jossey-Bass, San Francisco.

Lazarus, R. (1980) 'The stress and coping paradigm', in L. Bond and J. Rosen (eds) *Competence and Coping During Adulthood*, University Press of New England, Hanover.

Lesemann, F. (1981) *Du pain et des services; la réforme de la santé au Québec*, Editions St-Martin, Montréal.

Lincoln, Y. (1990) 'The Paradigm Revolution, Fourth Generation Evaluation and Health Promotion', (keynote paper, First National Conference on Health Promotion Research), Centre for Health Promotion, University of Toronto.

Lifman, M. (1978) *Power For the Poor – Family Centre Project: An Experience in Self-Help?* George Allen & Unwin, London.

Lundberg, B. and Starrin, B. (1990) 'Fighting health hazards at work: experiences from participatory research on workplace related health issues', (Research Report No 1), Centre for Public Health Research, Karlstad.

Lyotard, J. F. (1984) *The Postmodern Condition: A Report on Knowledge*, translated by G. Bennington and B. Massumi, Manchester University Press, Manchester.

McEwen, E. D. (1979) 'Mais qu'est-il donc arrivé au rapport Lalonde?', *Canadian Journal of Public Health* 70: 16–20.

Mackenzie, S. (1988) 'Balancing our space and time; the impact of women's organisation on the British city, 1920–1980', J. Campling (ed.) *Women in Cities, Gender and the Urban Environment*, Macmillan, Hampshire.

McKeown, T. (1971) 'An historical appraisal of the medical task', *Medical History and Medical Care*, Oxford University Press, Oxford.

—— (1976) *The Role of Medicine: Dream, Mirage, Nemesis?* Nuffield Provincial Hospital Trust, London.

McKnight, J. (1985) Keynote address: Regenerating Community in Proceedings, 'Empowerment through Partnership' Conference, Ottawa. Canadian Mental Health Association.

McQueen, D. V. (1989) 'Thoughts on the ideological origins of health promotion', *Health Promotion* 4: 339–42.

Manning, N. (ed.) (1985) *Social Problems and Welfare Ideology*, Gower, London.

Manson-Willms, S. (ed) (1992) *Building Bridges for Health Promotion Research*, Institute for Health Promotion Research, University of British Columbia, Vancouver.

Marlin, J. *et al.* (1983) *The Book of American City Rankings*, New York, Facts on File Publications.

Martin, C. J., Platt, S. and Hunt, S. M. (1987) 'Housing conditions and ill health', *British Medical Journal* 294: 1125–7.

Mays, N. (1990) 'Recent changes and developments in Department of Health research management', *Medical Sociology News* 16: 28–35.

Milio, N. (1986) 'Multisectoral policy and health promotion: Where to begin?', *Health Promotion* 1: 129–32.

Mitchell, S. C. and Davies, J. K. (1985) 'The use of the media in health education

– a view of its evolution in Scotland', in D. S. Leathar *et al.* (eds) *Health Education and the Media II*, Pergamon Press, Oxford.

National Civic League (1991) *Healthy Communities Initiative Update*, The National Civic League, Denver, Colorado.

Newby, N., Nowotny, H., Alsop, A. and Smith, J. (1991) 'Social sciences in the context of the European Communities', (European Science Foundation/Economic and Social Research Council report).

Nutbeam, D. (1986) 'Health Promotion glossary', *Health Promotion* 1: 113–27.

Nutbeam, D. and Catford, J. (1987) 'The Welsh heart programme evaluation strategy: progress, plans and possibilities', *Health Promotion* 2: 5–18.

Oliver, M. (1992) 'Changing the social relations of research production', *Disability, Handicap and Society* 7: 101–14.

O'Neill, M. (1989) 'The Political Dimensions of Health Promotion Work', in C. Martin and D. V. McQueen (eds) *Readings for the New Public Health*, University of Edinburgh Press, Edinburgh.

—— (1990) 'Healthy Cities indicators; a few lessons to learn from Europe', in J. Feather and B. Mathur (eds) (1990) *Indicators for Healthy Communities* (proceedings of an invitational workshop; Saskatoon, Health Status Research Unit, Department of Community Health and Epidemiology, University of Saskatchewan, pp. 33–8.

O'Neill, M. and Cardinal, L. (eds) (1992) *Des indicateurs pour évaluer les projets québécois de Villes et villages en santé: la nécessité de faire des choix*; Groupe de recherche ét d'intervention en promotion de la santé de l'Université Laval (GRIPSUL), DSC de l'Hôpital de l'Enfant Jésus et DSC de l'Hôpital St-Sacrement, Québec.

O'Neill, M., Cardinal, L., Fortin, J. P., and Groleau, G. (1990) 'La naissance du réseau québécois de Villes et villages en santé', *Recherches Sociographiques* 31: 405–18.

OPCS (1986) *Registrar General's Decennial Supplement on Occupational Mortality 1979–85*, HMSO, London.

Orr, J. (ed.) (1987) *Women's Health in the Community*, Wiley, Chichester.

Owen, A. and Mohr, R. (1986) 'Commentary: politics and pitfalls in evaluation', *Community Health Studies* 10: 95–9.

Patton, M. (1986) *Utilization – Focused Evaluation*, Sage, Beverly Hills.

Parfitt, J. (1987) *The Health of a City: Oxford, 1770–1974*, The Amate Press, Oxford.

Pederson, A., Edwards, R., Kelner, M., Marshall, V., and Allison, K. (1988) *Co-ordination de la politique publique favorisant la santé*; Santé et Bien-être Social Canada; Direction de la Promotion de la santé, Ottawa / *Co-ordinating Healthy Public Policy: An Analytic Literature Review and Bibliography,* Ottawa, Health and Welfare Canada, Health Services and Promotion Branch Working Paper No. HSPB 88 – 1.

Planned Approach to Community Health (PATCH). Reference Manual: Facilitator's Guide and Co-ordinator's Guide, (November 1989), Centres for Disease Control, Atlanta, Georgia.

Platt, S., Martin, C. J. and, Hunt, S. M. (1989) 'Damp housing, mould growth and symptomatic health state', *British Medical Journal* 298: 1673–8.

Prout, A. (1990) *MESMAC Evaluation, Illumination, collaboration, facilitation, negotiation – evaluating the MESMAC project.* Health Education Authority, London.

Rathwell, T. (1991) 'Too many bits and pieces', *The Health Service Journal*; 14 March: 22–3.

Reich, M. and Goldman, R. (1984) 'Italian occupational health: concepts, conflicts, implications', *American Journal of Public Health* 74: 1031–41.

Renaud, M. (1981) 'Les réformes québécoises de la santé ou les aventures d'un état narcissique', in L. Bozzini *et al.* (eds) *Médecine et Société*, Editions St-Martin, Montréal: 513–51.

Research Unit in Health and Behavioural Change, (RUHBC) (1989) *Changing the Public Health*, Wiley, Chichester.

Richardson, A., Jackson, C. and Sykes, W. (1990) *Taking Research Seriously, means of improving and assessing the use and dissemination of research*, Department of Health, HMSO, London.

Rifkin, S. B. (1981) 'The role of the public in the planning, management and evaluation of health activities and programmes, including self-care', *Social Science and Medicine* 15: 377–86.

Rootman, I. (1988) 'Le développement des connaissances; un défi pour la promotion de la santé', *Health Promotion/Promotion de la santé* 27: 2–4.

—— (1989) 'Knowledge for health promotion; a summary of Canadian literature reviews', *Health Promotion International*; 4: 67–72.

Rosen, G. (1979) 'The evolution of social medicine' In H. E. Freeman *et al.* (eds) *Handbook of Medical Sociology*, Prentice Hall, Englewood Cliffs, New Jersey.

Ross, E. (1991) 'The Origins of Public Health', in P. Draper (ed.) *Health through Public Policy*, Green Print, London.

Sainsbury, P. (1991) 'Neighbourhood Watch', *Nursing Times* 87: 66–8.

Sandercock, L. (1978) 'Citizen participation: the new conservative', in P. N. Troy (ed.) *Federal Power in Australia's Cities*, Hale and Iremonger, New York.

Schutz, A. (1967) *The Phenomenology of the Social World*, North Western University Press, Evanston.

Schwartz, N. B. (1982) 'Anthropological views of community and community development', *Human Organisation* 40: 313–22.

Sherwood, D. (1991) personal communication to M. O'Neill.

Shustermann, R. (1988) 'Post-modernist aestheticism : a new moral philosophy', *Theory, Culture and Society* 5: 337–55.

Smith G. and Cantley, C. (1985) *Assessing Health Care*, Open University Press, Milton Keynes.

Smith, S. J. (1989) 'Housing and health: a review and research agenda?', Discussion Paper No. 27, Centre for Housing Research, Glasgow University.

Smithies, J. (1991) 'Management Development and Community Development', (paper presented at the Open University/HEA Roots and Branches Winter School, Open University.

South Australian Health Commission (1988) *A Social Health Strategy for South Australia*, S. A. Health Commission, Adelaide.

Southern Community Health Research Unit (1989) *Measuring the Health of the City*, South Australian Health Commission, Adelaide.

—— (1991) *Planning Health Communities: A Guide to doing community needs assessment*, South Australian Health Commission, Adelaide.

Southern Community Health Services Research Unit (1987) *Which Way to Go? A*

Study of Community Health Centres in the Southern Metropolitan Area of Adelaide, Southern Community Health Services Research Unit, S. A. Health Commission, Adelaide.

—— (1988) *Where Are We Going? A Restudy of Community Health Centres in the Southern Metropolitan Area of Adelaide*, Southern Community Health Services Research Unit, S. A. Health Commission, Adelaide.

Stake, R. E. (1967) 'The countenance of educational evaluation', *Teachers College Records* 68: 523–44.

Starrin, B. and Lundberg, B. (1990) 'Participatory research: a 1990's challenge for the emancipation of working-life research', Paper presented to the conference on Work and Welfare, University of Karlstad, Sweden, 17–20 June, 1990.

Stevenson, H. M. and Burke, M. (1991) 'Bureaucratic logic in new social movement clothing: the limits of health promotion', *Health Promotion International* 6: 281–91.

Stirling, A. (1991) personal communication to M. O'Neill.

Strong, P. M. (1986) 'A new-modelled medicine? comments on the WHO's regional strategy for Europe', *Social Science and Medicine* 22: 193–9.

Szaz, T. (1972) *The Myth of Mental Illness : Foundations of a Theory of Personal Conduct*, Paladin, London.

Thomas, P. (1986) 'The use of social research: myths and models', in M. Bulmer (ed.) *Social Science and Social Policy*, Allen & Unwin, London.

Thunhurst, C. (1989) 'Towards a Core Set of Indicators', Core Indicators Group, Report to the UK Healthy Cities Network, Liverpool.

Tones, K., Tilford, S. and Robinson, Y. (1990) *Health Education: Effectiveness and Efficiency*, Chapman and Hall, London.

Traynor, M. (1990) *Measuring the Health of the City: A glimpse of the invisible Christie Downs*, Southern Community Health Research Unit, Adelaide.

Tsouros, A. (1990a) 'Healthy Cities means community action', *Health Promotion International* 5: 177–8.

—— (ed.) (1990b) *World Health Organisation Healthy Cities Project: A Project Becomes a Movement (Review of Progress 1987 to 1990)*, WHO/FADL, Copenhagen.

Wadsworth, Y. (1984) *Do-it-yourself Social Research*, Victorian Council of Social Services, Melbourne.

—— (1988) *Participatory Research and Development in Primary Health Care by Community Groups*, (Consumers Health Forum, Canberra, February).

—— (1991) *Everyday Evaluation on the Run*, Action Research Issues Association, Melbourne.

Webster, C. (1990) *The Victorian Public Health Legacy: A Challenge to the Future*, Institute of Environmental Health Officers/Public Health Alliance, Birmingham.

Weiner, C. (1980) *The Politics of Alcoholism*, Transaction Press, New Jersey.

Weiss, C. (1986) 'The many meanings of research utilization', in M. Bulmer (ed.) *Social Science and Social Policy*, Allen & Unwin.

Whitehead, M. (1988) *The Health Divide*, Penguin, London.

WHO (1946) *Constitution*, World Health Organisation, New York.

—— (1978) *Primary Health Care: A Report on the Conference on Primary Care (Alma-Ata)*, WHO, Geneva.

—— (1984) 'Concepts and Principles of Health Promotion', a Discussion Paper, WHO/Euro, Copenhagen.

—— (1985) 'Research in health promotion: priorities, strategies, barriers', report of a joint WHO/SHEG workshop held in Edinburgh in November 1984, WHO Euro, Copenhagen.

—— (1986) 'The Ottawa Charter for Health Promotion', WHO, Canadian Public Health Association, Health and Welfare Canada, Ottawa.

—— (1986b) 'Notes of Healthy Cities Planning Meeting', Copenhagen 13–17 January 1986, unpublished paper.

WHO Healthy Cities Project (1988a) *Promoting Health in the Urban Context*, WHO Healthy Cities Paper No. 1, FADL, Copenhagen.

—— (1988b) *Five-Year Planning Framework*, WHO Healthy Cities Paper No. 2, FADL, Copenhagen.

—— (1988c) *A Guide to Assessing Healthy Cities*, WHO Healthy Cities Paper No. 3, FADL, Copenhagen.

Wilkins, R. and Adams, O. (1983) *Healthfulness of Life*, Institute for Research on Public Policy, Montreal.

Winter, R. (1987) *Action-Research and the Nature of Social Injury*, Professional Innovation and Education Work, Avebury Brookfield, Vermont.

Wohl, A. S. (1983) *Endangered Lives : Public Health in Victorian Britain*, Dent, London.

Worsley, T. (1990) *National Evaluation of Health Cities Australia Pilot Project*, Australian Community Health Association, Sydney.

Zander, L. *et al.* (1989) 'Statement from the Association of DH/DSS – funded research workers on the DH/DSS contract of research', *Medical Sociology News* 15: 222–4.

Ziglio, E. (1988) *Trends in Canadian Health Policy: Before and After the Lalonde Report*, RUHBC, Edinburgh.

Index